Pandemic Minds

Praise for *Pandemic Minds: COVID-19 and Mental Health in Hong Kong*

'The almost three-year-long COVID-19 pandemic was difficult for many, especially amongst low-income families. We are still suffering from the long COVID of mental health. Mental wellness of the population during COVID-19, particularly amongst those who had been quarantined, was overlooked by authorities. *Pandemic Minds* provides many insights to prevent repeating mistakes again.'

—**Paul S.F. Yip**, director, Centre for Suicide Research and Prevention, University of Hong Kong

'*Pandemic Minds* is a vital and telling book, with moving stories of the huge impact of COVID-19 on people in Hong Kong. This book also offers the prospect of a silver lining from this collective disaster, namely that it is now more possible to speak about mental health problems, and that COVID-19 may in fact have helped to reduce mental health stigma.'

—**Sir Graham Thornicroft**, professor of community psychiatry, King's College London

'A thoughtful and well-researched account of the many different facets of the COVID-19 pandemic in Hong Kong. Kate Whitehead's engaging narrative and case studies bring back to life memories of a time that challenged the mental health and well-being of so many of us and will help us all to reflect upon and learn from the experiences that we shared.'

—**Hannah Reidy**, clinical psychologist

'*Pandemic Minds* delves into the profound psychological aftermath of the global crisis and how it has reshaped our understanding of community and mental health care. This book is an essential blueprint for anyone committed to the cause of mental health in a post-pandemic world that will resonate with readers long after the last page is turned.'

—**Candice Powell**, CEO, Mind HK

'The Hong Kong COVID-19 response was characterised by a top-down, disease-based approach with little thought given to psychological and social well-being. The power of this book lies in the individual narratives. I would encourage anyone with an interest in those times to take a walk in some other Hong Kong shoes.'

—**David Owens**, honorary clinical assistant professor in family medicine, University of Hong Kong

Pandemic Minds

COVID-19 and Mental Health in Hong Kong

Kate Whitehead

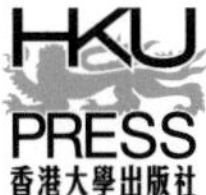

Hong Kong University Press
The University of Hong Kong
Pok Fu Lam Road
Hong Kong
https://hkupress.hku.hk

ISBN 978-988-8842-89-6 (*Paperback*)

British Library Cataloguing-in-Publication Data
A catalogue record for this book is available from the British Library.

Digitally printed

Dedicated to the resilient people of my beloved home, Hong Kong

Contents

Acknowledgements

The value of this book lies in the honesty and authenticity of the stories it tells. I begin by expressing my gratitude to everyone who generously shared their experiences. Some chose to be named, while others opted for pseudonyms—all of you are equally brave and generous for stepping forward to speak your truth.

Many individuals played a crucial role in connecting me to a diverse range of people: Aaron Busch kindly spread my initial call out for first-hand accounts of the pandemic on his @tripperhead X account; Stephanie Law (Culture Homes) immediately understood the project and offered assistance; Jeff Rotmeyer and Roni Li (ImpactHK) introduced me to members of their community and assisted with translation; Raymond Yang at Just Feel provided a safe space for some individuals in his network to share their story; Father John Wotherspoon (Mercy HK) invited me to Sunday lunch at his Temple Street chapel, where I met some of his congregation, Surdham Lam (Flow Bookshop) connected me to frontline medical workers; and Amanda Li (StoryTaler) and the team at MIND HK helped spread the word.

Thank you to my good friends and first readers: Professor Yeewan Koon provided shrewd and humorous feedback on the first few chapters; and Dr Judy Blaine read each chapter and offered thoughtful comments. Special thanks to Sarah Stewart and Peter Parks at Agence France-Presse for securing fantastic images for the book. And let's not forget my Wordle-loving sister, Sue Leaver, who came up with the snappy title.

A heartful appreciation to everyone at Hong Kong University Press who provided invaluable support: Michael Duckworth quickly embraced the idea of this book; Yasmine Hung helped navigate readers' reports and gather endorsements; and the copyediting and production team was ever patient and supportive.

Finally, sincere thanks to all those friends who offered unwavering support and encouragement: Cathy Hilburn Chan, Palani Mohan, Johan Nylander, Catherine Platt, Rachel Smith, my sister Sam Thomas, Bettina Wassener, and Kim Wedderburn.

1

Introduction

As COVID-19 spread across the globe, it took the lives of millions of people. Technology and social media at our fingertips, we watched in real time as countries scrambled to respond to this unprecedented crisis. But there was no playbook for a pandemic of this scale, and governments were forced to prioritise physical health above all else. Yet, as the months wore on, it became clear that the virus was taking a toll on our mental well-being too. According to the World Health Organization (WHO), rates of anxiety and depression surged globally by 25 percent in just the first year of the pandemic (WHOa, 2022).

Hong Kong's battle with COVID-19 was a gruelling one. The first case was reported on January 23, 2020, and the government swiftly implemented measures such as social distancing, mask mandates, cross-border travel bans, and mandatory quarantine regulations. For two years, these efforts kept the virus at bay. However, in March 2022, Hong Kong was hit hard. The financial district's streets were deserted, restaurants and bars were closed, and supermarket shelves were empty. Many elderly residents remained unvaccinated, and the city recorded the highest number of COVID-19 deaths per capita globally.

The WHO defines mental health as 'a state of mental well-being that enables people to cope with the stresses of life, realise their abilities, learn well and work well, and contribute to their community' (WHOc, 2022). Yet for many in Hong Kong, the pressure of prolonged isolation, repeated school closures, business closures, job losses, and the ever-present fear of infection severely challenged their mental well-being. The tension on the street was palpable, as masked people hurried to and from home. Tempers flared on short fuses. As the demand for mental health care surged, the public mental health care system buckled under the pressure. Patients faced years-long waits for an initial consultation.

In March 2022, a study by the mental health charity Mind HK found that 38 percent of respondents reported their mental health had worsened in the preceding two months. Almost half (49.9 percent) showed symptoms of mild to severe depression, and 41.3 percent showed symptoms of mild to severe anxiety (Mind HK, 2022).

It wasn't until a year later, on March 1, 2023, that the city's three-year mask mandate was finally lifted. But many people continued to wear face masks in public. Officially, the pandemic was over, but the mood on the street didn't match the government's HK$100 million 'Hello Hong Kong' campaign to welcome back tourists.

Rather than rising phoenix-like from the ashes, Hong Kong emerged battered and bruised. The city was still reeling from the 2019 protests when the three-year pandemic hit. Businesses closed, more than 200,000 people left—the biggest population drop in more than 60 years—and many were struggling financially. Hong Kong needed time to recover from a tumultuous four years.

Mental health professionals had been warning of a looming crisis for years. The signs were there: a surge in suicides, studies revealing alarming levels of anxiety and depression throughout the city. Yet it was only after the mask mandate was lifted that the true extent of the crisis became apparent. In a series of shocking incidents that shook the city to its core, a wave of violent stabbings left residents reeling. On June 2, 2023, a man with a history of mental illness fatally stabbed two women at a shopping mall. Just a week later, another man attacked a woman near an MTR station, leaving her with serious injuries. And on June 18, a 29-year-old McDonald's worker was arrested after he assaulted his store manager with two knives following an argument about his work performance. As people laid flowers for the victims, calls grew for an overhaul of the city's mental health services and greater support for those in need.

This book delves deeper than the cold, hard data found in scholarly articles about the toll of the pandemic on mental well-being in Hong Kong. With compassion and curiosity, it seeks to reveal the human side of the crisis. Rather than pointing fingers at the government's policies, it serves as a record of Hong Kong's journey, for future reference. For those still grappling with the aftermath, it offers a chance for reflection and healing, providing both a sense of solidarity and practical tools for coping. By going beyond the numbers, we can glean insights from a city that endured one of the longest COVID-19 pandemic periods and be better prepared for whatever may come next.

One of the positive outcomes of the pandemic is that it's brought mental health to the forefront of public conversation. While there is still a stigma about mental health in Hong Kong, perceptions are slowly changing, and it is becoming more acceptable to discuss these issues openly.

This book presents a rich tapestry of perspectives, of both men and women of all ages and socio-economic backgrounds. While the majority of narratives come from Hong Kong Chinese residents, reflecting the local population, the experiences of eight other nationalities are also represented for a more inclusive picture. These accounts are genuine and told in the individuals' own voices. To foster candour, contributors were given the choice to use their full name, first name, or a pseudonym, as indicated at the beginning of each section.

Speaking openly about mental health takes courage, and I'm grateful to those who shared their personal stories for this book. They did so in the knowledge that their experiences could help others. When we are open about our struggles, it makes it easier for others to come forward. Many of those interviewed said that talking about their experiences helped them process what had happened, and for some, reflecting on those tumultuous years allowed them to reframe their experiences. One pilot even reached out after the interview to say that sharing his story gave him the courage to seek counselling. Such is the power of voicing your struggles and being heard. Though the stories are personal and specific to Hong Kong, the emotions they invoke are universal, and the insights on mental health can be applied worldwide.

The pandemic laid bare a stark divide between the haves and have-nots in Hong Kong. Those with means were able to weather the storm with relative ease, buoyed by their resources. They transitioned to remote work, ensconced in spacious homes that accommodated comfortable work and study set-ups. They could afford extended hotel quarantines and travelled when the rest of the world opened up. And if they needed mental health support, private therapy was readily available. That is not to say the affluent were immune to mental health struggles—far from it—but the odds were tipped in their favour.

But for the working class, especially those in manual labour and the service industry, the pandemic brought job losses and financial insecurity. Many lacked savings to fall back on and were forced to endure cramped living conditions that strained family relationships. Those who sought mental health support through the public system faced a daunting 40-month waiting list.

As a mental health counsellor during the pandemic, I saw mostly clients who were fortunate enough to afford private practice fees. Many had never experienced mental health issues and were alarmed at how the prolonged disruptions were affecting their well-being. There was an increase in anxiety and stress-related issues, and some people were struggling with panic attacks for the first time. As the pandemic continued, mental health and relationship challenges stemming from stress, fear, anger, and loneliness became more common. Without intervention, early symptoms can escalate to depression and PTSD and lead to substance abuse.

I provided support to cargo pilots who were struggling with the intense pressure of their airline's demanding closed loop system, which kept them away from home and loved ones for six-week stretches. These men, accustomed to maintaining emotional control and clear thinking in crises, were now pushed to their limits.

In mid-2022, I saw the growing demand for mental health services and decided to offer *pro bono* counselling at a community centre for migrant domestic workers. This was a group with no access to mental health support. These women faced high levels of stress, primarily due to financial concerns and worries about their families back home. Despite their incredible resilience, they were in urgent need of emotional support.

I also taught small groups Trauma and Tension Releasing Exercises (TRE) to help them better self-regulate and manage stress. Some clients used TRE to cope with the three-week hotel quarantine. While none of the individuals who shared their stories for this book were my clients, my professional experience undoubtedly influenced the content.

I have called Hong Kong my home since the age of seven. Through the good years and the bad, my love for this vibrant metropolis has never faltered. I bore witness to the SARS epidemic as a staff member of the *South China Morning Post*, when overnight, everyone donned masks and touched elevator buttons with their elbows, fearful of a mystery virus. I was in Hong Kong through the COVID-19 years, save for three fraught trips to the UK to support a family member. Those return journeys ended with extended hotel quarantines. I got through them by employing all the strategies I'd been advising my clients to use to maintain good mental well-being during self-isolation.

In an ideal world, mental health support would be within everyone's reach. Regrettably, that's not the reality we live in. Lengthy wait times in the public system deter many from seeking help, and private therapy is often prohibitively expensive. But there are things we can do to take care of our mental health daily. It's just as important as physical fitness and health.

At the end of each chapter are healthy coping skills and strategies designed to help manage distress and tackle problems before they become overwhelming. Mental health isn't static; it can change over time, with periods of stability and difficulty. By talking openly about it, we make it easier to seek help when we need it. Therapy isn't just for those who are struggling; it's for anyone who wants to improve their mental well-being.

2

Quarantine

In Hong Kong, the mandatory three-week quarantine was an overriding feature of the city's pandemic response. While elsewhere in the world isolation was mostly done at home, in this city of 7.4 million people it largely took place in purpose-built government facilities or, for those returning from overseas, at designated quarantine hotels. But in a city where space is at a premium, the average hotel room, just like the average flat, is small. Most of the quarantine hotel windows didn't open, leaving residents to endure three weeks without fresh air. And stepping foot outside your quarantine room was made a criminal offence, a poster on the back of every door detailing the punishment—a maximum fine of HK$25,000 and six months imprisonment.

***Siu-hang** (not her real name) was 22 weeks pregnant when she returned to Hong Kong from a business trip in July 2022. Her husband and two-and-a-half-year-old daughter were both at home. She tested positive for COVID-19 on her second day in a quarantine hotel.*

'When they told me I was positive, I didn't know how to handle the situation because I was pregnant. I thought I should see a doctor, so they sent me to hospital. I got to the hospital at about 6 pm and they put me in an isolation room by myself. It was freezing in there, and I was really uncomfortable and waited a long time to see a doctor. The whole time I was in hospital I felt really anxious; I didn't know what was happening. When I eventually saw a doctor, in the early hours of the morning, he said, "This is a virus; there's no medication." They said they were sending me to Penny's Bay. I asked if I could go to a [government quarantine] hotel instead, but they said only women 26 weeks pregnant or more could go to the hotel. At 4 am, I was put in a minivan with other people. It was so late, and I was so tired; it was crazy.

'When I arrived at Penny's Bay, they gave me a WhatsApp number to call if I needed anything and an alarm to activate in case of emergency. Dinner was given at 6 pm and breakfast at 8 am. On the second day, they forgot to give me dinner. I had gestational diabetes and was really hungry. I messaged the WhatsApp number and spent ages going through a series of automated messages: "Is this your first message? What do you want? Please wait for staff to contact you." But no staff followed up. I wanted to speak to a human, but it was impossible. I put a sign on my door saying, "Pregnant woman; needs to eat". I saw a "white soldier" [staff in white hazmat suit] walk past, and I opened the window and shouted out, "I haven't had dinner." The white soldier spoke to the robot, but he didn't get a response either. Everything there was automated.

'I was feeling really helpless, anxious, and stressed. I kept messaging and getting no reply. By 9 pm, I was starving; I hadn't eaten since lunch at noon. I saw another white soldier and called out the window again. He said the kitchen was closed, but he could give me instant noodles. I said I was pregnant; I couldn't eat instant noodles. He said he couldn't help and walked away. I was angry. I wanted to eat a nutritious meal for my baby. If I could have opened the door, I could have gone to a restaurant, but I was locked up in there. I felt it was now an emergency, so I pressed the alarm. Nothing happened; no one came. The red button was supposed to be the last resort, but it didn't work.

'I started thinking if I can't even get food, what would happen if I had a problem with my pregnancy? What if I started bleeding? I couldn't sleep and my fears were escalating. I needed to protect my baby. I called my husband and he found the email for the head of the Centre for Health Protection online. I emailed him at 4 am, telling him, "If I can't get dinner, which is a small thing, what if I can't get medical help when I need it?" I made it clear; I'm not pinning the blame on anyone. I want to be collaborative; I just want a solution. I didn't feel safe at Penny's Bay. I wanted to be in a place where I could get an ambulance if I needed it. If I'd been able to speak to a human, I don't think my fears would have escalated like they did.

'My email worked, and someone from the Hospital Authority called me at 10 am. I was so grateful that a real person responded and talked to me. I was moved to a quarantine hotel at 6 pm the next day. When I got to the hotel, I realised it was only half full. I don't know why they hadn't sent me there in the first place. It took 10 days before I got a negative result and I was released. Normally, I'm very co-operative. I support the Hong Kong government, but could they not take mercy on a pregnant woman?

'If you can complain in a rational way you can get help, but you have to know how to do it. What about the people who don't know how to express themselves like that to get their needs met and to be safe? I was very unhappy. Being fed is such a basic need. I appreciate the efficiency of Hong Kong, but everything was very bureaucratic; it lacked the human element.'

In April 2021, ***Brenda Adrian****'s mother passed away suddenly in her native Germany. She flew to Germany and helped her father arrange the funeral and returned on May 7 to begin her three-week hotel quarantine.*

'I didn't have the time to mourn my mother while I was in Germany because I was so busy arranging things and supporting my dad. The whole bureaucracy was a nightmare and my personal needs were pushed aside. I was running like a chicken with my dad and then I had to return to Hong Kong for my job and the three-week quarantine. No direct flights were available, and I had to go via Doha. I had to board the flight to Hong Kong within 48 hours of my negative COVID test result. It was so stressful getting the documents ready for my return.

'My mother's death hit me on the flight back, when I had time to think. Being pushed into that hotel room was horrible. I sat there for a long time. My mind was like a blender; I didn't have any clear thoughts. I'd done a two-week quarantine the year before, but then my mindset was totally different. That time, I went in thinking I'd get over my jetlag and have some time to do something for myself. But this time my mind was scrambled. I hadn't had time to mourn. But how could I mourn when there was no one there for me? There was no shoulder to lean on. It was brutal.

'There was no reason to get out of bed. I felt like crying but sat there numb. I was literally numb—it was like waking up from anaesthesia. I cried a lot. It was the whole situation. You ask yourself, "Where are you these days? What's the meaning of life?" I've never been like that. I had so much time on my hands and began searching online for the phases and symptoms of someone dying. I kept thinking that if I'd known all that, I would have made it back to see my mum one more time.

'The day after I arrived, the government reduced quarantine from three weeks to two. I called the government hotline several times to see if I could be let out after two weeks. Each time they said they'd call back but never did. I was desperate and called the German consulate, and they checked and said I'd have to stay the full three weeks even though people arriving after me were being released earlier. I understand they had to draw the line somewhere, but I really wanted to get out. I'd been away so long that I needed to physically be with someone to help deal with how I was feeling.

'Two days before I was released, I had my final PCR test. The result was to be given the next day. The wait was unbearable. A normal mind would say, "You've been in here for 20 days; there is no way you will test positive." But because I'd been in there so long and quarantine was messing with my rational thinking, I wasn't thinking clearly and was so worried. When I eventually received my negative result, I had a total breakdown. I cried non-stop for 20 minutes and kept checking the message.

'A three-week quarantine in a normal mindset is hard enough, but when you have a special burden like I had it's different. My partner said when I was released from quarantine, I was different. I was quieter and more serious and didn't crack jokes like I usually do. It took about six weeks before I started acting more like my normal self.'

Sarah *(not her real name) is in her 30s. In March 2021, her boss went to Ursus Fitness, a gym in Sai Ying Pun district, before work and was unknowingly infected with the virus. After working out, he went to* *the office and two days later tested positive for COVID-19. Sarah and her colleagues were considered close contacts and sent to Penny's Bay Quarantine Centre.*

'We got a call from the government to tell us that we were close contacts. They told us to stay at home and be on standby to be taken to a facility in a couple of days. The timeline was pretty vague. I was a little freaked out because no one really knew what was going on. I asked if I needed to prepare anything, but I didn't get an answer. I'm on a plant-based diet, so I didn't know what to expect with regard to food. I overpacked and brought two or three bags with me and my yoga mat.

'I was taken to Penny's Bay. I was pleased to see the room was pretty spacious and there was hot water, but the mattress was terrible, and the food was horrific. I did a PCR test and the following day they said I was positive, and I'd be picked up in an hour. I'd only just made a nest for myself and had to pack up all my stuff.

'I was taken by ambulance to a makeshift hospital somewhere on Lantau. The nurse asked what happened, and I said I'd got COVID at the office. She said, "Why didn't you wear a mask?" That passing comment really upset me. I'd just tested positive; I was in hospital and didn't know what was going to happen. I didn't need to be reprimanded. It was a lack of soft skills.

'There were two people in the ward when I arrived, and two more arrived the following day. We were all women and quite a young group working in hospitality, banking, and the media. It was 16 degrees Celsius in the room. I was wearing leggings, the hospital pants and shirt, a sweater, and woolly socks. And still I was freezing. Putting us in a highly air-conditioned area probably delayed our recovery. We all wanted hot water to warm up, but they wouldn't give it to us. The best they would do was microwave a plastic bottle of water. The water was barely warm, and we wondered about microplastics in it. We kept asking for a kettle, but they wouldn't allow it. Someone in another ward managed to smuggle in a folding kettle, but it was confiscated. It would have been fine if they had given us hot water.

'The hospital staff were stretched very thin, and we contacted them by pressing a buzzer by the bed and then someone came to the ward. They could see us through the glass, and we communicated on a phone. It took us three days to work out how to adjust the bed so that we could sit up more easily during the day. My boss and colleagues gave me their blessing not to work, but I did. It was good to have a distraction.

'Aside from the cold, the main issue was the lack of preparedness and information. We had no idea what the test criteria were to be released. They came in hazmat suits and gave us regular blood tests and chest X-rays, but we didn't know what they were looking for. It was hard to get any information. In the end, we got information through the Ursus WhatsApp group. Everyone was sharing information about what to do; it was a great support system.

'Meals were delivered through an air-locked compartment. The food was edible; some dishes were bland, but some were tasty. I was lucky to be on a ward where everyone was friendly and helpful and checked in on each other. One by one, the others were released, and I was the last one. Because it was just me on the ward, they moved me to another ward where everyone had their curtains drawn around their bed. It was an extremely uncomfortable atmosphere. I didn't know when I'd be released and was starting to lose hope.

'I had lots of blood tests. Perhaps because the staff were overworked and tired, they didn't always get the needle in right. When I left, I was so bruised I had the arms of a heroin addict. I wouldn't wish that experience on anyone. It was traumatic; a very difficult time. The trauma was more about the mistreatment and anger at the government for how everything was handled. I was down for quite a little while after I was released. It was tough mentally, but then I got the hang of it. We set up a group chat with those people who were on the ward, and we get in touch once in a while. Sometimes, I'll run into one of them on the street and we give each other a hug. It was such an extreme experience, like living in a dystopia.'

Kelvin *(not his real name) is in his 20s and has lived at Kwai Chung Estate in Kwai Tsing district with his parents since he was five years old. In January 2022, two blocks of the public housing estate were subjected to a seven-day lockdown after 20 COVID-19 cases were detected. Kelvin and his family were among the residents forced to home quarantine in their 300-square-foot flat.*

'When I came home from work, I was shocked to see more than 30 police and government officials outside my building. They were setting up metal crowd-control barriers and told us we needed to do a PCR test. It wasn't very organised. People were scrambling to do the test as fast as possible and get home. The scariest part was stepping outside the front door. I went downstairs with my mum and dad. We were wearing N95 masks, face shields, and gloves. We queued for an hour to do the test. It felt like a risk standing there with so many people, and we cleaned ourselves with alcohol as soon as we got back home.

'We were allowed out the next morning. At work, a friend of a friend told me that the government was thinking of doing a complete lockdown on my building. I called my parents, and we hurried to the supermarket to stock up. We'd heard about Wuhan and Shanghai lockdowns and how people suffered because they couldn't get enough food, so we prepared for the worst and bought lots of meat and vegetables. Each block is 14 floors high, and there are 20 flats per floor. We are friendly with the neighbours opposite and next door, so my mum WhatsApped them and suggested they also stock up on food.

'We were worried about all the unknowns. What was going to happen to us in the next few days? Would we get the virus? We knew if we got infected, we'd be sent to a quarantine facility, and those places didn't have a good reputation. On the third day, they announced a complete lockdown and said we needed to do a daily PCR test. The government officials got better about organising the testing, so it wasn't as chaotic as the first few days. There were rumours that we would be sent to a quarantine facility, which was our biggest fear, because the environment there is not good. But the government worked out that there weren't enough rooms in the facility to house us all, so they asked us to stay in our own flats.

'Five police officers were posted outside the entrance to our building, and another five guarded the exit. It would have been impossible to leave. We felt isolated from the rest of the world. During that time our bond with our neighbours was strong because we were all in same boat. I was lucky that I could work from home. I had a good relationship with my colleagues, and they FaceTimed me in their lunch break, which gave me something of a social life. Many people living in housing estates have less secure jobs; they are paid by the hour or the day, and some lost their jobs because they could be easily replaced.

'Mental health during a lockdown depends a lot on whether you get enough personal space in your flat. Hong Kong flats are much smaller than flats in other countries, which can lead to a high-pressure life. My relationship with my parents is okay—not too good, but not too bad. We had some conflicts, mostly related to daily chores like the washing and the laundry. Our neighbours, also in a 300-square-foot flat, are a family of five. They sleep in bunkbeds and have even less personal space than us. If you have many conflicts with family members and have to stay with them for a week or more, you can imagine how tense it can get. When I opened my window, I often heard arguments breaking out among my neighbours. Some people really shouted and used foul language.

'In the first few days, the government gave each flat some cleaning products and groceries. After a few days, we were given soup and some fruit. The food was about as good as you'd expect in a *cha chaan teng* [tea restaurant], and in the final few days we took the free meals and didn't cook. Because Chinese New Year was coming, we were given canned abalone and a box of cookies. The food and groceries were probably worth about HK$1,000. The media coverage of our estate was intense, so the government knew if they delivered low-quality groceries it would damage their reputation. Once we got over the shock and fear of the lockdown, my parents and I felt okay. We were fed regularly and given free resources. Aside from the fear of getting infected, which didn't go away, things got better.

'We found out from the news that the lockdown on our estate was ending. We received a letter thanking us for our cooperation from the government. We had mixed feelings about that because we hadn't a choice but to cooperate, but I suppose a letter was better than nothing. Chinese New Year was immediately after the lockdown, but we didn't visit our relatives for fear of getting infected. We decided to play it safe and stay at home. At the time, we thought that lockdown was bad, but the fifth wave which followed in March was much worse.'

***Jean-Paul** (not his real name) is a successful business executive in his early 50s. He spent the first year of the pandemic with his wife and children in Hong Kong. In the spring of 2021, he had to take a business trip, which meant undergoing a three-week hotel quarantine on his return. He'd never experienced a mental health issue, and the period in solitary confinement left him shaken.*

'I had to travel for business, which meant I had to do the three-week hotel quarantine. I wasn't looking forward to it, but I wasn't worried. I thought it would be okay if I was prepared and thought about how I would spend my time in quarantine.

'Twenty-one days is a long time to spend in one room, so I paid the extra money and got a good hotel on the south side with a sea view. The hotel was not too far from my home, which was strange. I packed a bag of books to read, and my wife delivered it to the hotel, along with my guitar. I thought finally I would have some time to learn to play.

'I'd read a book about a French nun who spent decades living as a hermit. I knew from her experience that if you want to stay sane you must have a routine, so that was my plan. I was disciplined in the first week and kept to my plan.

'I didn't spend much time reading the books because I was spending so much time looking out to sea at the ships. There are many ships crossing the Lamma Channel. I wondered where they were going. I ordered binoculars so I could read the names of the ships and then looked them up online to see where they were sailing. It became so important to know where they were going. After a while, I began recognising the ships. When you have zero contact, it makes a difference when you see a ship that you saw a few days before. It almost feels like a friend.

'I spoke to my family on the phone, but it wasn't the same as speaking to them face to face. My first real conversation was on day 10. There was knock on the door, and there were two men in hazmat suits. One of them said in an aggressive tone, "Sit in that chair; give us your passport." Imagine: I've not spoken to anyone for 10 days and this is what I hear? I know they were there to do a job, and it must be hard doing all those PCR tests, but if he'd said, "Hello, how are you doing?", it would have made such a difference.

'It takes determination and willpower to stick to your routine and not let yourself drift. After two weeks I'd had enough. I was exhausted. The last week was horrible; I woke up twice in the morning in tears. Imagine—you wake up and you are crying. It was frightening. My expectation was that when I entered the final stretch I'd be fuelled by new energy, which didn't happen. Maybe that's why I was broken.

'When I was released, I thought I'd want to see friends and go out and in the fresh air, but I found I didn't want to. I had invitations for the weekend, but I turned them down. I needed some time to adjust to life outside. The quarantine was much harder than I expected it to be.'

* * *

The psychological impact of quarantine can be far-reaching and long-lasting. Research shows that the negative mental health outcomes of quarantine can range from low mood, irritability, exhaustion, and insomnia to confusion, anger, and post-traumatic stress symptoms. And the longer the duration of social isolation, the greater the risk of poorer mental health outcomes (Brooks et al., 2020). Hong Kong's three-week hotel quarantine was one of the longest COVID-19 quarantines in the world.

On February 8, 2020, Hong Kong implemented its first compulsory quarantine for people entering from mainland China. But as the pandemic spread, the policy evolved. Starting from March 19, all travellers arriving from overseas were required to undergo a 14-day compulsory quarantine at home or in other accommodation of their choice. To reduce contact between travellers from overseas and the local community, the government mandated that arrivals from high-risk places must quarantine at hotels, starting on July 25. And in December of that year, the compulsory quarantine was extended to three weeks for almost all international travellers. But as the pandemic began to recede, the policy shifted once again. In early 2022, the quarantine duration was reduced to two weeks and then to one week, the policy finally concluding at the end of September that year.

As social creatures, humans are naturally inclined towards social interaction. But when subjected to social deprivation for 21 days, our inherent nature is put to the test. Research has shown that quarantine periods of just one to three days have no negative mental health effects (Wassenberg et al., 2010). However, when the isolation period reaches the one-week mark, adverse mental health outcomes begin to appear. A study conducted in the US showed significant negative alterations in mood and anxiety after only one week of isolation (Catalano et al., 2003). And another study found that people who were isolated for two weeks due to contact with MERS patients suffered from high rates of anxiety and anger, the poor mental health effects persisting even four to six months after their release (Jeong et al., 2016).

In the wake of Hong Kong's quarantine, two peer-reviewed studies have delved into its impact on mental health. The first, a qualitative study conducted in 2021 by Dr Judith Blaine, revealed that many individuals who underwent quarantine experienced feelings of isolation, confinement, loneliness, anger, depression, and anxiety. These individuals reported lingering physical effects such as back problems, muscle aches, and brain fog. However, more commonly reported were lingering feelings of fear, anxiety, anger, exhaustion, lack of energy, and difficulty with social integration. Months after quarantine, some individuals were still experiencing PTSD, depression, and insomnia. Others expressed feelings of anger and resentment towards policymakers for imposing this 'punishment' on them. For most participants in the study, it was the lack of openness and transparency that created the adverse psychosocial effects.

In 2022, a study conducted by Hazan and Chan in Hong Kong examined the mental health outcomes of 248 people undergoing either a two-week or a three-week quarantine. The study found that depressive symptoms peaked in the second week of quarantine. Several predictors of worse mental health outcomes were identified, including poor sleep, a lower sense of meaning, and a longer duration of quarantine.

Interestingly, the study also considered the effect of indirect contact with nature. The results showed that individuals with rooms that had a view of green spaces fared better than those without such a view. The authors suggested that the natural environment may act as a buffer against some of the negative impacts of quarantine. However, the opportunity to select a room overlooking nature was only available to those in hotel quarantine. Furthermore, these rooms were priced at a premium, costing upwards of HK$1,200 per night. As such, this option was only accessible to the wealthy.

A three-week quarantine can be challenging even for individuals with good mental health. However, for those with a history of poor mental health or who are experiencing a difficult life event, such as the death of a loved one or a divorce, the experience can be particularly difficult. The social support that would typically help them through tough times, such as a hug from a loved one or a chat with a close friend over a cup of tea, is not possible during quarantine. Without the opportunity to emotionally regulate with another person, these individuals may experience a rapid decline in their mental health.

Australia adopted a progressive approach to quarantine, screening individuals before they entered quarantine. Those deemed at risk or in need of additional support were assigned to a different type of accommodation, such as a flat with windows that could be opened and from which knives had been removed. Additionally, everyone in quarantine received a daily phone call from the government to check on their well-being and ask how they were coping.

In contrast, Hong Kong implemented a one-size-fits-all quarantine policy and no screening to identify individuals who might be vulnerable or at risk. Once the quarantine door was shut, the only person those in isolation saw was a PRC tester, whose job was to quickly and efficiently administer a COVID-19 test. Dressed in full-body biohazard suits, these testers did not inquire about the general well-being of those in quarantine and adhered to a strict and formal script, using only the words necessary to perform their duty: 'Open the door, sit on the chair, open your mouth.'

These testers could have been empowered to ask individuals how they were doing. This simple act could have provided a means of identifying those who were struggling and allowed mental health professionals to follow up with a phone call and offer psychological support if necessary.

Returning to Hong Kong was an expensive and stressful endeavour due to regular flight cancellations and a shortage of quarantine hotels. However, those who chose to return and undergo quarantine still had the advantage of agency, as they ultimately made the decision to return. In contrast, individuals entering a government isolation facility did not have this choice. People sent to a purpose-built facility, either because they had tested positive for COVID-19 or were a close contact of someone who had, received little prior notice and had no say in where they were sent.

Penny's Bay Quarantine Centre, located on Lantau Island, was the largest government facility for quarantine in Hong Kong. The sprawling camp opened in July 2020 and accommodated 270,000 people over its two and a half years of operation. Initially, the facility housed close contacts of COVID-19 patients but later transitioned into housing for confirmed COVID-19 cases.

In late February 2022, during the peak of the Hong Kong pandemic, Penny's Bay housed 8,000 people. This period, known as the 'fifth wave', marked the camp's darkest period. As COVID-19 swept across the city, fear of being taken to Penny's Bay far outstripped concerns over the virus itself. People were terrified of being separated from their families and were often admitted to the camp in a state of high anxiety.

As the number of individuals in the camp swelled, bottlenecks in the testing system emerged. Some individuals who had completed their 21 days of isolation were still waiting for their test results before they could be released. During this period, one man broke quarantine rules and slept outside his isolation unit to protest a lack of support in obtaining urgent medication for a chronic condition. In the midst of this chaos, there were four reported suicide attempts within a 27-hour period (Whitehead, 2022).

As the pressure reached boiling point, 16 people at the camp staged a walkout due to a lack of clear instructions on when they would be released. A viral video on Facebook showed a visibly distressed woman arguing with security guards. Her clothes and hair were dishevelled, and she shouted, 'Don't pretend to care about me! I want to go back! I have recovered! I'm crazy!' Many people at the camp witnessed the woman's emotional breakdown, but no one came forward to support her, presumably out of fear of being punished for breaking the rules of their internment. The guards, who might have comforted her, were unable to handle the situation and called the police when she lashed out at one of them. The climate of fear surrounding the virus and the need to be seen following strict regulations meant that when the police arrived, they failed to recognise that this was a woman in extreme emotional distress. Her case was logged as assault occasioning actual bodily harm. The video is still available on the online platform Reddit. Many of those who commented on the video questioned whether Hong Kong had become tunnel-visioned in its pursuit of protecting people from the virus, losing sight of its humanity in the process.

Some people have likened Penny's Bay to a prison, surveillance cameras installed outside every room and reprimands issued from loudspeakers if anyone set foot outside or even opened the door (Paul, 2021). Common complaints about the camp include the lack of Wi-Fi, poor-quality meals, and unclear information. These are all recognised as critical stressors during quarantine that can have a negative impact mental on health. Research has shown that the ability to activate one's social network and communicate with family and friends is essential in reducing feelings of isolation, distress, and panic (Brooks et al., 2020). The inability to do so can not only create immediate anxiety but also lead to longer-term distress.

The study by Brooks emphasises the importance of having a phone or online service staffed by healthcare workers to provide clear instructions to those in quarantine and to show that their needs are recognised and they have not been forgotten. Although a hotline was set up for those in government isolation facilities, there were widespread complaints that it was understaffed (Heung & Lam, 2022). The hours spent on hold and waiting for calls to be returned only added to the sense of frustration.

Many expatriates turned to the English-language HK Quarantine Support Group, a Facebook community that offered crowd-sourced advice, up-to-date information, and a sympathetic ear. People went to it for advice on quarantine regulations and food delivery services, as well as a platform to rant about injustices and hardships. Some members even offered support and advice to those suffering panic attacks and claustrophobia in isolation. The group quickly gained recognition as not only a major source of information but also a source of comfort and solidarity, growing quickly from 30,000 members in February 2021 to more than 95,000 by the end of 2022. Feeling connected to others through a shared experience can be validating and empowering, offering people the support they may not be getting elsewhere (Pan et al., 2005). Feeling heard and connected to society is integral to mental health during quarantine, and the HK Quarantine Support Group played a key role in making many feel included (Blaine, 2021).

Some people were fortunate enough to be able to work while in quarantine, which not only ensured a steady income but provided them with a focus and sense of purpose while in isolation. However, for those who couldn't bring their work with them, such as manual labourers and those in the service industry, an unexpected stint in quarantine created significant financial pressure. A 2022 poll by the Democratic Alliance for the Betterment and Progress of Hong Kong found that 39 percent of those surveyed had been forced to take unpaid time off for their compulsory isolation period, and 57 percent reported losing income as a result of their diagnosis (Ma,

2022). Financial loss due to quarantine has been shown to create serious socio-economic distress, which is a risk factor for psychological disorders, anger, and anxiety several months after quarantine (Brooks et al., 2020).

Mandatory quarantine without public discussion can have a negative impact on mental health. Blaine (2021) suggests that allowing people to feel heard and have a sense of autonomy can reduce these consequences. Instead of enforcing quarantine, Blaine proposes relying on altruism to mitigate the mental health impact. She emphasises the importance of balancing public safety with human rights and calls for inclusiveness, reasonableness, openness, and transparency when making decisions about quarantine measures.

In Blaine's study, participants proposed several ways in which policymakers could support the mental health of those in quarantine. These include shortening the duration of quarantine, allowing people to quarantine at home, providing access to fresh air and exercise opportunities, serving decent food, permitting people to leave their homes once a day, and offering professionally staffed telephone support lines available 24/7 (Blaine, 2021).

Strategies and Support / Seven-Step Quarantine Survival Guide

1. Be well prepared. Good preparation is essential. If you are going to a government isolation facility, you are allowed to bring in as much as you can carry. If you are returning from overseas and it's a planned quarantine, you'll have plenty of time to prepare. Consider packing a case in advance and asking a friend to drop it off at the quarantine hotel. In addition to clean clothes and toiletries, bring healthy food and snacks. Think about how you will want to spend your time and bring the things you'll need for those activities, whether it's work, reading, learning a language, or taking an online course. It is worth thinking about who you might call if you are struggling and what you will do to manage stress. A few creature comforts, such as a favourite blanket, pillow, or framed photo of a loved one, will help you settle in and feel at home.

2. Take ownership of your room. As soon as you move in, unpack and organise the room in a way that suits you. This might mean moving the furniture, perhaps pushing the bed against the wall to create more space to exercise, or moving the desk to the window. Find a place to store your luggage so that it's out of sight, and put personal items in drawers. An uncluttered room will feel more spacious and will help you stay focused and productive.

3. Keep to a daily routine. Creating a structure and sticking to it is the golden rule of quarantine. You will be entirely responsible for the rhythm of your days, and if you don't establish a routine at the outset, you risk sliding into a murky void of time which can make quarantine feel even longer. Critically, decide what time you are going to get up, set an alarm, and stick to it. Get showered and dressed, and after breakfast, engage in the goals that you've set yourself, whether it's working, studying, or doing in a creative project. It is important to set yourself breaks, avoid screens before you go to bed, and turn the lights out at the same time each night, because getting a good night's sleep is essential for mental well-being. Take it easy at the weekend and give yourself a chance to rest and recharge, ready for another week.

4. Stay physically active. It is essential to engage in some form of physical activity every day, ideally 30 minutes of vigorous exercise. If you don't already have a daily exercise routine, go online and find one that suits; take it as an opportunity to try something new. You could even put on your favourite music and dance. Physical activity reduces levels of cortisol and adrenaline, the body's stress hormones, and helps to reduce anxiety.

5. Stay connected. Human connection is essential for our mental health. Having at least 30 minutes a day communicating with friends or family will serve as a buffer from feelings of isolation or disconnection. The real benefits are to be had speaking directly to someone, either on a video platform or the phone rather than texting. This will be a critical part of your mental wellness in quarantine, so it is worth setting up the calls in advance, perhaps organising a virtual group gathering or reaching out to reconnect with old friends.

6. Be kind. Firstly, be kind to yourself. Quarantine is a very challenging situation, and it's important to recognise that and accept that not everything will go perfectly. If you are having a bad day and not able to keep to your routine, that's okay. Consider what will help you move out of a rut, whether it's speaking to friend, exercising, or getting lost in a book. Although you may feel alone, there are many people around you—someone in the room next door, someone delivering your meals, or the testing staff. Try showing small acts of kindness, whether it's a pleasant word to the PCR tester or sending a note to someone you know who might be struggling in quarantine. Research shows that people who engage in regular acts of random kindness see a boost in their happiness levels.

7. Get help if you need it. Long periods in isolation can leave us with plenty of time to ruminate. Dwelling on bad memories, regrets, or past choices can lead to overthinking, and anxieties can escalate. This can be especially difficult for people in isolation following a recent challenging life event, such as the death of a loved one or a divorce. If you feel overwhelmed or are having thoughts about hurting yourself, help is available even in isolation.

The Samaritans 24-hour telephone hotline / +852 2896 0000
The Samaritan Befrienders Hong Kong / +852 2839 2222
Suicide Prevention Services (24 hour) / +852 2382 0000

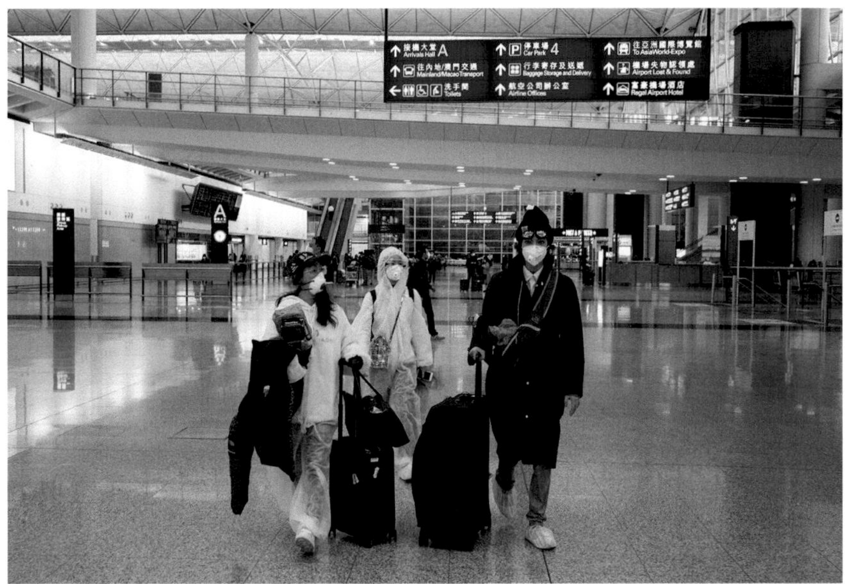

Passengers wearing protective gear, as a precautionary measure against COVID-19, walked through the arrivals area after landing at the Hong Kong International Airport on March 18, 2020. The following day all travellers arriving from overseas were required to undergo a 14-day compulsory quarantine. Photo by Alastair Pike © AFP.

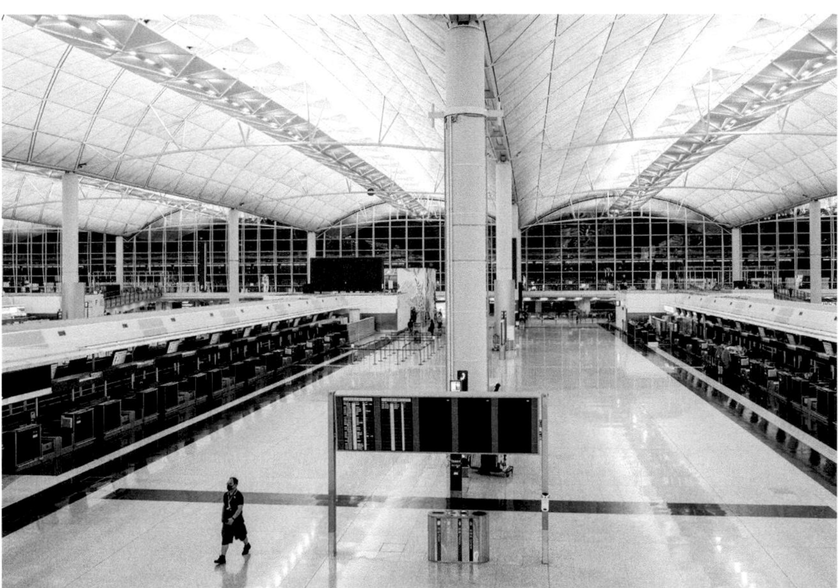

Hong Kong International Airport was deserted on March 24, 2020, hours before a ban on all non-residents from entering the city from midnight in a bid to halt the spread of the virus. Photo by Anthony Wallace © AFP.

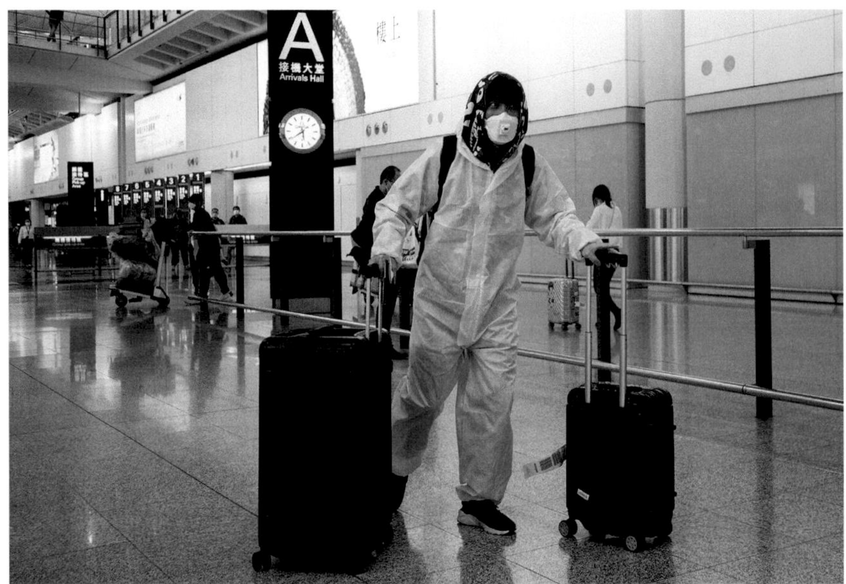

In 2020, Hong Kong International Airport experienced significant declines due to the impact of COVID-19. The airport handled 8.8 million passengers and 160,655 flights, representing year-on-year decreases of 87.7 percent and 61.7 percent, respectively. Photo by Alastair Pike ©AFP.

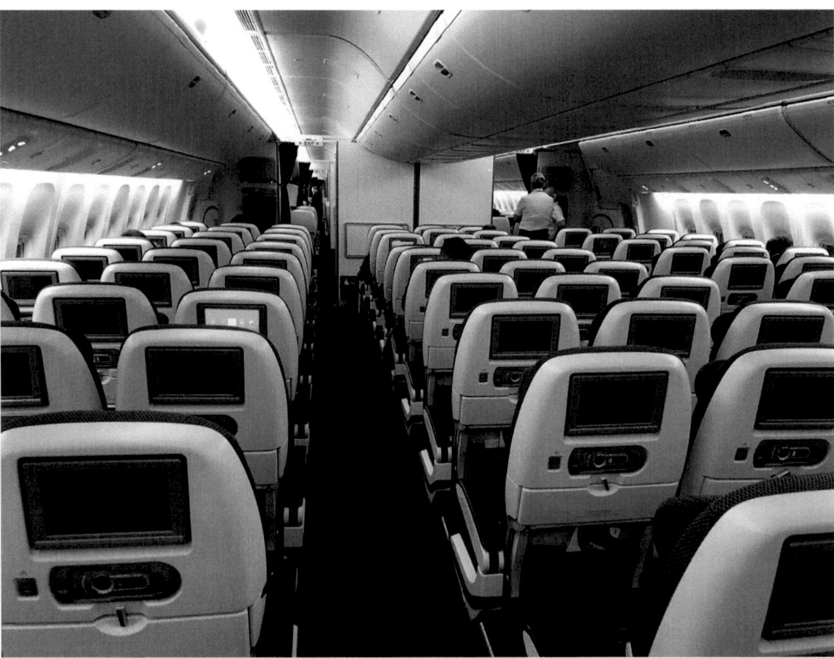

A nearly empty Cathay Pacific flight in April 2020. The introduction of a compulsory two-week hotel quarantine, which was extended to three weeks in December 2020 for almost all international travellers, severely reduced travel to Hong Kong. Photo by Kate Whitehead.

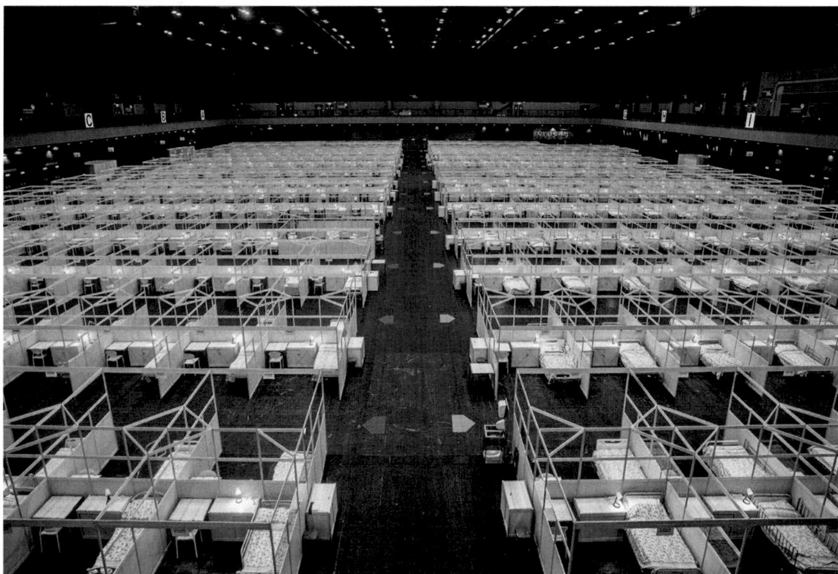

This 500-bed temporary field hospital at Asia World Expo opened on August 1, 2020 to accommodate stable COVID-19 patients as the city saw new wave of virus outbreak and postponed its legislative elections citing public health reason. Photo by Isaac Lawrence © AFP.

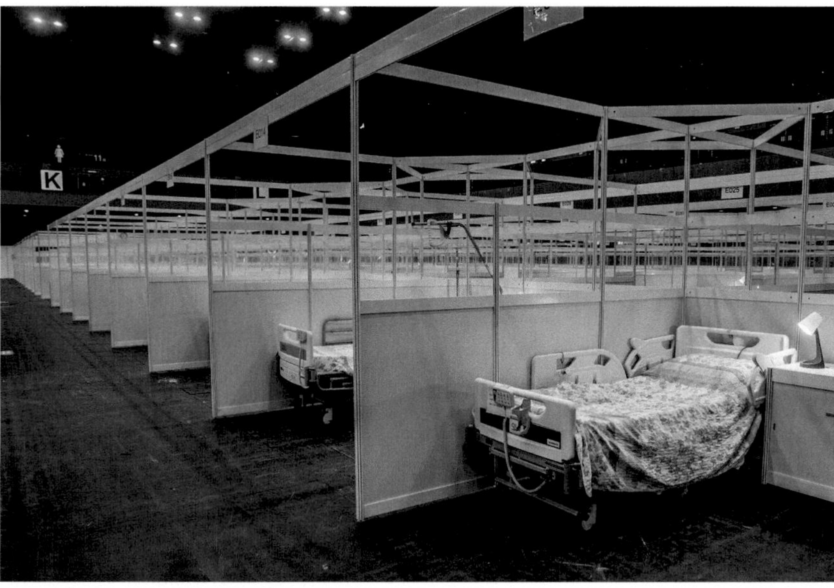

The opening of the temporary field hospital at Asia World Expo came a day after Chief Executive Carrie Lam announced the postponement of upcoming legislative elections for a year, saying that the decision was to protect public health and had 'nothing to do with politics'. Photo by Isaac Lawrence © AFP.

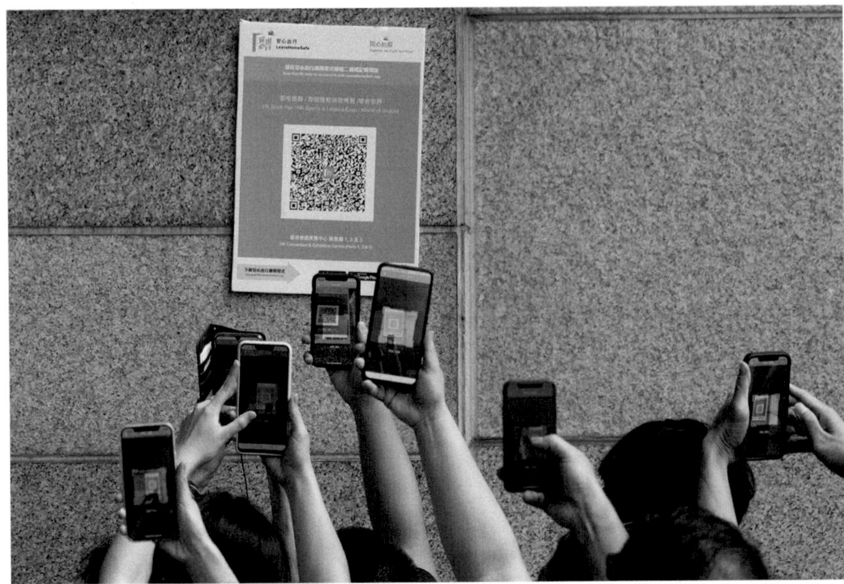

Visitors scanned a QR code for the Hong Kong government's 'Leave Home Safe' app to trace people in the advent of any COVID-19 outbreaks, as they queued up to enter the annual Hong Kong Book Fair in Hong Kong on July 17, 2021. Photo by Bertha Wang © AFP.

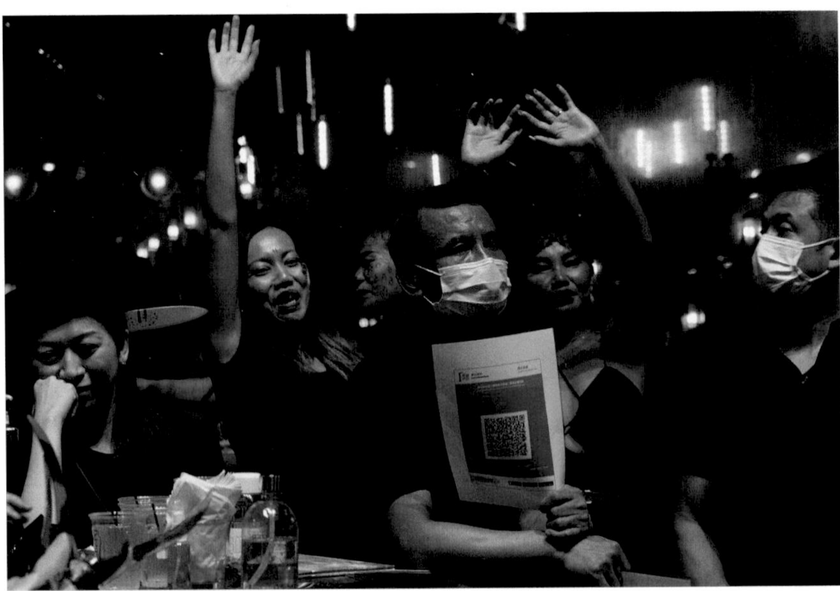

On Halloween night 2021, a man tried to ensure that the revellers in a Lan Kwai Fong bar had registered with the Hong Kong government's 'Leave Home Safe' app designed to trace people in the advent of a COVID-19 outbreak. Photo by Bertha Wang © AFP.

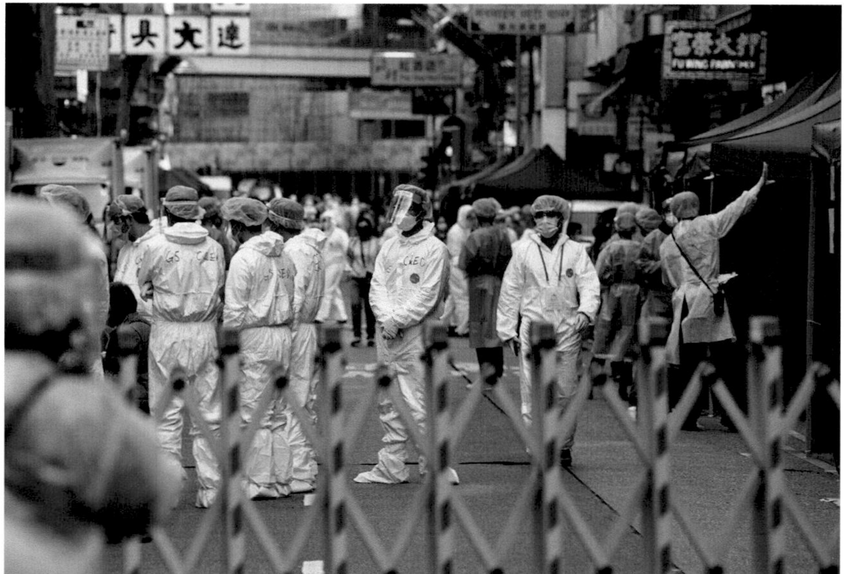

Health workers conducted testing in Jordan on January 23, 2021, after thousands were ordered to stay in their homes for the city's first COVID-19 coronavirus lockdown as authorities battle an outbreak in one of its poorest and most densely packed districts. Photo by Peter Parks © AFP.

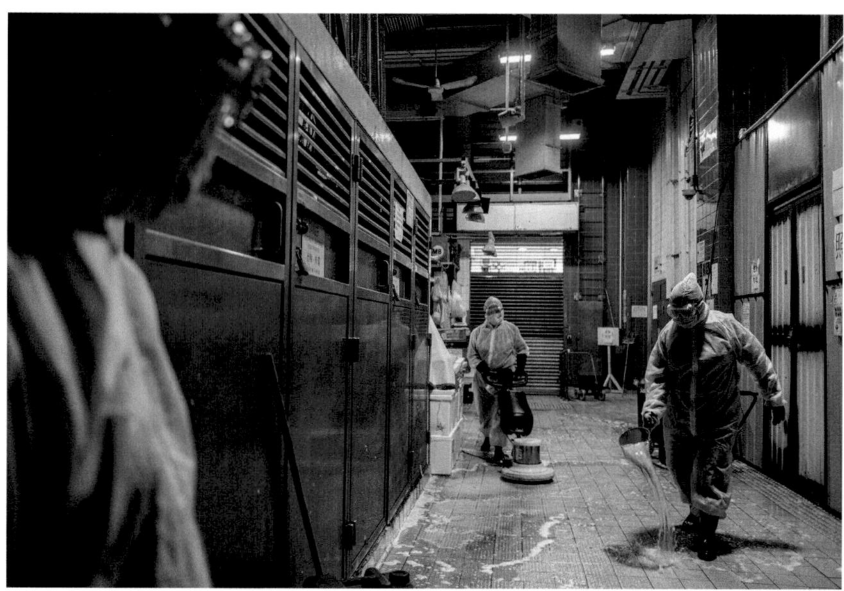

Food and Environmental Hygiene Department contractors took part in a cleaning and disinfection of Pei Ho Street Market in Sham Shui Po days after Hong Kong reimposed tough social distancing measures on July 15, 2020, shuttering many businesses and making facemasks on public transport mandatory. Photo by Anthony Wallace © AFP.

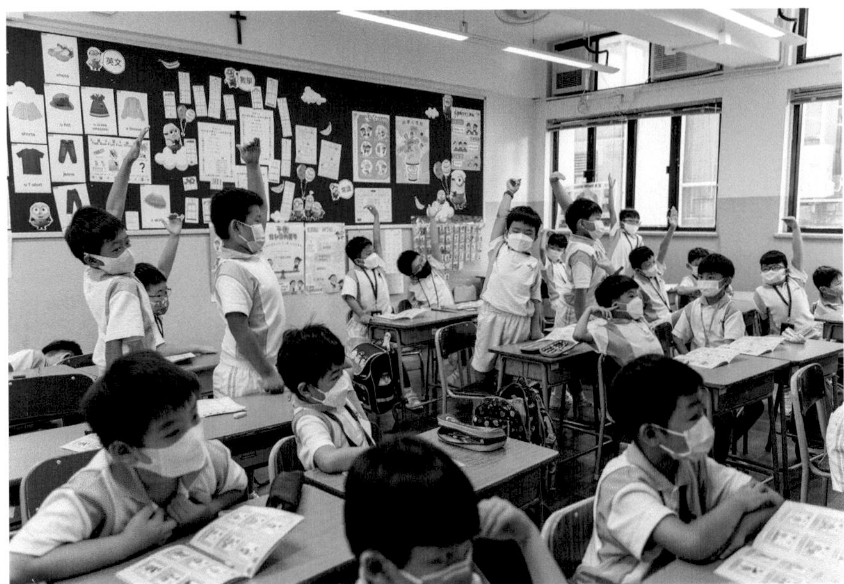

The extended duration of the mask mandate left its mark on many children and was most obviously seen in their speech development. Children learn pronunciation and phonics by watching and imitating the mouth movement of other people, which was not possible when everyone was wearing a face mask. Photo by Just Feeling.

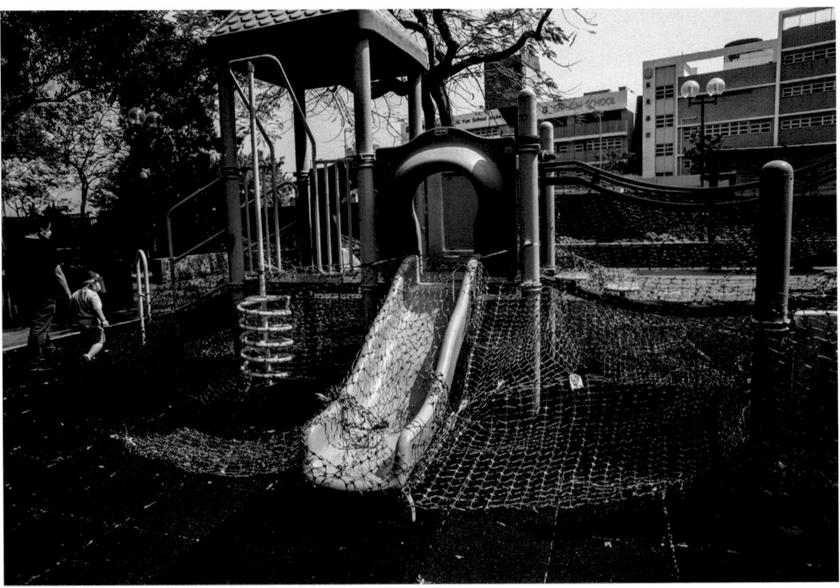

The impact of the pandemic was particularly hard on very young children who missed out on a proper kindergarten education and playdates. Outdoor playgrounds such as this one was fenced off to prevent children gathering and playing. Photo by Isaac Lawrence © AFP.

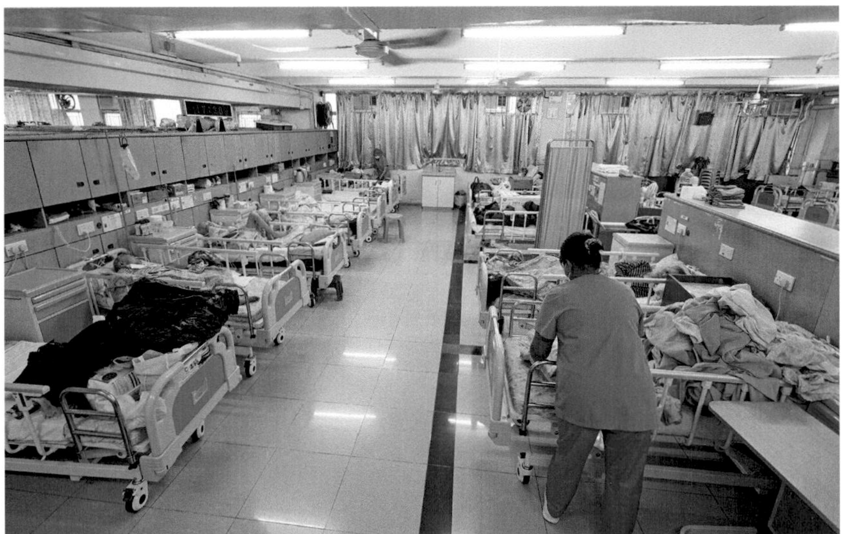

Staff tended to elderly residents at a care home. By June 2021, only 5 percent of 70- to 79-year-olds were vaccinated and just one percent of those over 80 had received the COVID-19 vaccination. Photo by Culture Homes.

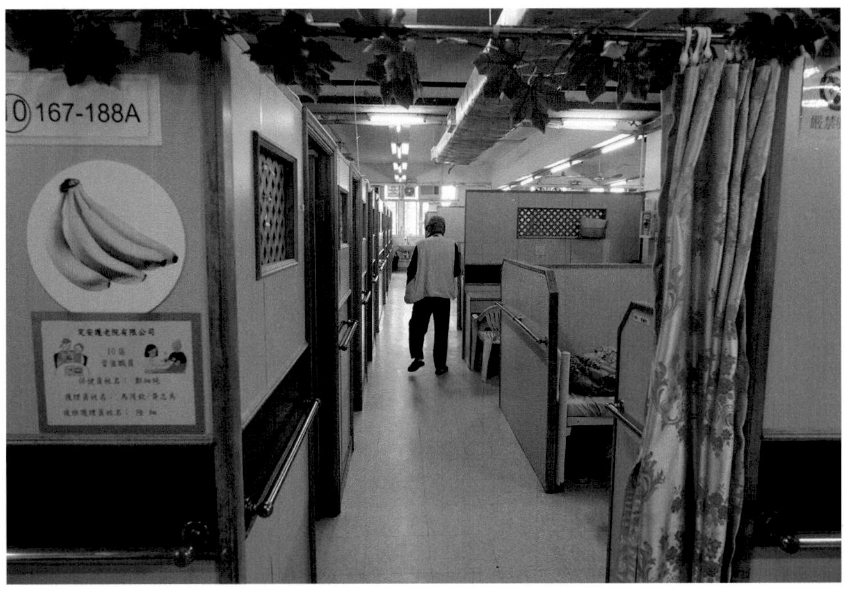

During the peak of the pandemic from February to May 2022, more than 9,000 people died and over 5,000 of them were unvaccinated elderly who were mostly in elderly care homes. Photo by Culture Homes.

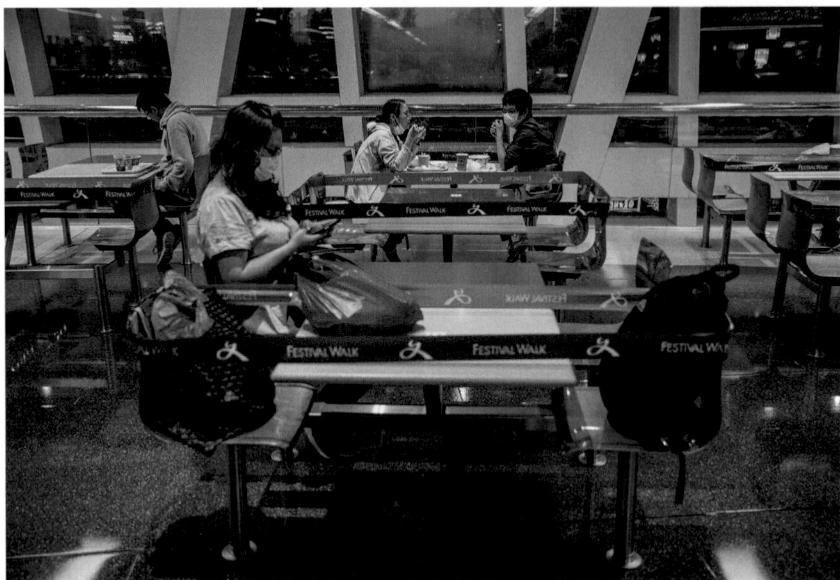

Social distancing measures meant restaurants only allowed tables for two people and closed at 6 pm. The strict regulations kept COVID-19 at bay, but they took their toll on people's mental health. Photo by Dale de la Rey © AFP.

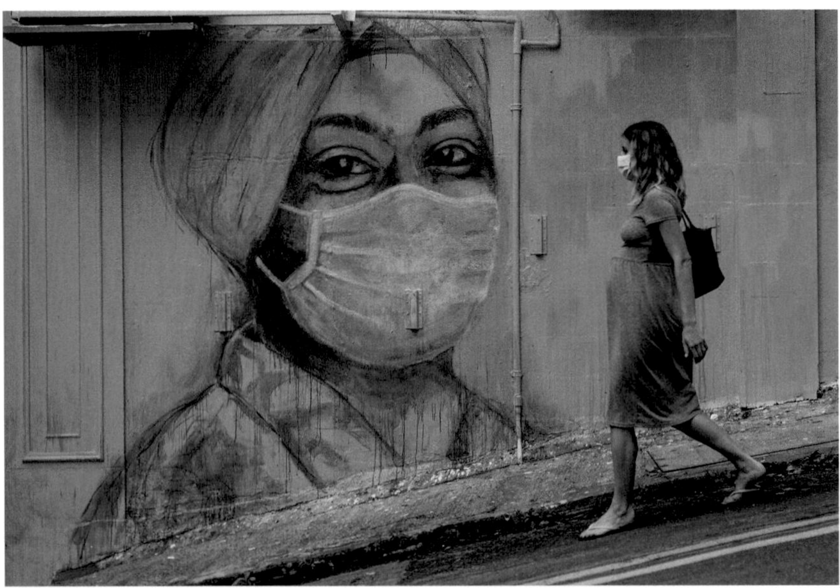

The pandemic introduced new challenges for expectant mothers: they were forced to navigate a world where antenatal exercise classes, seminars, hospital tours, and postnatal classes were all suspended and visits to mothers and babies staying in postnatal wards were not permitted. Photo by Anthony Wallace © AFP.

3

School Closures

Hong Kong was one of the first cities to mandate school closures during the pandemic. The four-month school shutdown in early 2020 was among the longest in the world. While other countries resumed face-to-face lessons or had hybrid classes, Hong Kong continued with the closures until mid-2022.

The impact of these closures was significant. In 2020, children in K1 to K3 went to school for only 30 to 50 days, instead of about 190 days before the pandemic. Primary school pupils had only 70 to 80 school days that year, and secondary students, 80 to 90 days. In 2021, schools mostly stayed closed for the first two months before students in different grades took turns to return. Half-day classes only resumed fully in late May. In January 2022, during the city's fifth wave of infections, classes were suspended, and the summer holiday was brought forward. Students only returned to school in batches in April and May (Yiu & Zhao, 2023).

The suspension of in-person classes and almost 450 days of school closures didn't just affect children's academic progress but also their mental health and social development. A year after the resumption of schooling, the lingering impact of months spent at home, isolated from their teachers and friends, is still being felt.

In 2020, **Marco** *was just three years old and had recently started attending a local kindergarten. However, due to the pandemic, his classes were held online via Zoom for almost two years. When we spoke to him in April 2022, two months after the mask mandate was lifted, he was six years old.*

'At the beginning [of the pandemic] I stayed at home. That made me happy, but then I felt sad because I couldn't go outside. I couldn't go to the park. I was bored at home and felt powerless. Then I got scared when we went outside. I didn't want to go outside because I didn't want people to look at me.

'I wore a mask for a really long time. It was very boring. I couldn't smell anything when I was wearing the mask, but it made me feel safe.

'When I went back to school it took me a long time to learn all my classmates' names. I have 23 classmates. I was happy to go to school because they have toys to play with. The teacher was wearing a mask, and she used a microphone so we could hear her. My classmates shouted because they were wearing masks. I didn't like it when it was so noisy, and everyone was shouting. Sometimes I saw someone at school not wearing a mask, and it made me really worried that I was going to get sick. I didn't like eating lunch at school because everyone took off their masks to eat and it made me scared.

'When they told us that we can take off our masks, I felt a bit terrified. But then I was happy. Now in my class there are 19 students not wearing a mask, and four of them are still wearing a mask.'

Marco's mother, **Chloe**, *also has a daughter named Leka. Leka was just one year old when the pandemic began. Chloe, who works as an HR executive, had to adapt to the new normal and work from home throughout the pandemic, while keeping an eye on her children.*

'The worst thing for the kids was that they needed to stay at home every day; they never went to the park. Imagine that—a three-year-old kid that never went to the park! As a parent, it was very stressful. We needed to follow the government policy, which changed from day to day. Sometimes it was about restaurants, sometimes it was about the masks, sometimes it was about work. During the day, I worked from home and delegated the online schooling to my domestic helper. After work, I needed to follow up on their homework and then check the government regulations to see if there was any update.

'In the first year, Marco had a 20-minute Zoom lesson once a day. The teacher wasn't experienced at running an online class and spent most of the lesson taking attendance. In the second year, the Zoom class was 20 minutes, a 15-minute break, and then another 20 minutes. By then, the teacher was better trained about how to run a Zoom class and knew how to mute everyone. The parents had to go to the school to collect the homework, and then the students had to show their homework on Zoom to the teacher. I don't think there was much learning happening at all. The teaching responsibility sat on the parents. It was a huge pressure. I didn't know how to teach them. I needed to work from home, so my domestic helper was the one sitting next to Marco for the online classes. It was a very stressful time. The kids were very noisy, and I was trying to work next door, which caused more stress. The online classes were in Chinese, and my domestic helper is from the Philippines and doesn't speak

Cantonese, so I had to run between rooms and try to follow the kids' schedule.

'I wasn't too worried about Marco academically because he was so young, but I worried about him missing out on the social life he should have been getting at kindergarten. After such a long period of social distancing, whenever we needed to leave the building Marco became afraid of people. He couldn't look at someone and say, "Hello". He didn't even want people to look at him, and he was afraid of coming across anyone outside our family. It became quite serious. If there was a neighbour beside the lift, he refused to leave the flat, and we had to wait for an empty lift.

'During this time, there were food scares, and I had to go to the supermarket to stock up. I tried to minimise the time that we went out. Marco wasn't afraid of COVID; he never got sick. What he became afraid of was seeing other people. The lack of social life and contact between people made him scared. My kids only saw me, my husband, and our helper. I tried not to go out at peak times because Marco would scream. He didn't know how to express the feeling that he was scared. If we were out and I saw people ahead of us, I'd slow down and give them time to move on.

'Because the kids stayed at home so much, they didn't develop strong muscles in their back, and their legs and were quite weak. Sometimes I had to take them to hospital for check-ups, just the standard check-ups that young kids need. Whenever we went to the hospital, I was very afraid of getting the virus and bringing the sickness home. Even when I was at home, I never felt very relaxed.

'Marco's Chinese language is not that good. After the first year of the pandemic, I took him to see a speech therapist. The therapist wore a face mask. When she was teaching Marco how to make the "s" sound, she found it hard to show him how to hold his tongue back without showing her mouth. Some months later, they introduced transparent face masks and she wore one of those, but it got fogged up. Marco got scared when he saw her mouth behind the plastic and asked her to wear the regular mask.

'The mask-wearing really affected his language learning. If the therapist hadn't been wearing a mask, Marco would have progressed much faster. I've been doing what I can to train him at home. I'm still taking him to speech therapy, and even now that they have lifted the mask mandate the therapist is still wearing a mask. She has the responsibility to keep every kid coming to the class safe. She doesn't want to get infected and pass it on, and she has her own family to think about as well.

'Leka is a COVID kid. She started wearing a mask when she was two years old. It was hard to find one to fit her little face. COVID babies know all the rules. She was our gatekeeper—if ever I forgot to wear a mask, she'd remind me. She was vigilant about obeying the rules. She always noticed the colour. When I changed from a blue to a pink mask, she was happy and pointed it out. When we sit down to eat, she immediately puts her hands out to ask for hand sanitiser.

'Leka started nursery school on Zoom when she was two years old. We had to buy her a school uniform and she put it on and sat in front of the screen. There were 20 students on Zoom. After a year of online nursery class, her first term of K1 was also at home. When she started going to real school she adapted quickly. At school, she knows when it is time to change to a new mask; she knows the schedule. Like I said, the COVID kids know all the rules.

'I encourage my kids to talk about their feelings every day. When Marco went back to school, he faced some challenges. In primary school, the boys can get a bit naughty. If someone is mean to him, he runs away; he doesn't know how to respond. Luckily, I have a good relationship with him, and he tells me what happened. Then I tell him a social story so he can better understand the situation and how to respond.'

***Winter** (not her real name) is a dedicated teacher in her late 20s. She teaches English to 10- to 12-year-olds at a local primary school in Kowloon. The majority of the students at her school come from low-income households.*

'At the start of the pandemic, when the schools were closed, the teachers were asked to record a video at home and send it to the students to watch. I made PowerPoint slides and recorded audio over the slides. I'm good with technology, so that was easy for me. Students could choose when to watch the video. There was no way of knowing if they had watched it, and I have no doubt there were some students who didn't watch it.

'The beginning of the pandemic wasn't too bad for me; I had a lot of free time. After six months our school began to do Zoom lessons. I hated that because I like to use a lot of body language when I teach, and I couldn't do that online. Not having face-to-face interaction with the students was hard.

'The students were trapped at home, and many had no one to monitor them. A lot of the time I felt I was talking to myself; I could tell from the movement of their eyes that they weren't focused on the lesson. There were definitely students who opened another window and were watching YouTube and not following the lesson.

'In the classroom, if students are reluctant to speak up, I will encourage them. But it was hard to do that on Zoom when you can't have eye contact. Lots of the students didn't want to share on Zoom; they didn't have the confidence. There were also technical problems.

Some students had poor Wi-Fi, and they would often drop out of the class and then log back in.

'My students are from low-income families, and often their parents couldn't help them when they were struggling with schoolwork. Those years of online schooling were very stressful. I knew the students weren't learning well, so there was stress in that. And sometimes their parents sat just out of view and watched the class, and I worried that if I made a mistake they might complain to the principal. That never happened, but it was still stressful knowing I was being watched by a parent.

'I heard that COVID was especially dangerous for elderly people, and I was worried about my parents. I asked them to stay at home and wear a mask. The Chinese media focused on the side effects of the vaccine, so we were afraid to get jabbed. My parents waited until the last possible moment, the point at which they wouldn't be able to go for dim sum if they weren't vaccinated. I also waited until they made it compulsory for teachers to be vaccinated.

'When in-person school restarted, the relationship between the students, teachers, and parents was poor. Many students hadn't learned anything during the pandemic, and everyone was stressed about their performance. There was a ton of homework that hadn't been done, and I had to keep asking the students and parents to finish it. I was concerned about them falling behind and stressed about getting them to quickly catch up. The parents were also pushing their kids. I think the pressure made the students more stressed and anxious. All of us, our well-being is poor even now. The relationship between the teachers and parents has deteriorated—it was all because of the COVID situation.

'It has been two months since the government dropped the face mask regulation, but some students are anxious about taking off their masks. They don't want to show their face. I see that especially with the older students, 11 to 12 years old. I don't wear a mask, but most of the teachers at school are still wearing a mask; only two or three are not. The ones who are wearing masks tell me they are afraid of getting COVID or the flu, especially those with young families at home.

'Some of my students are lagging behind in speech development. They ask silly questions and aren't as mature as the students I taught three years ago. They are stressed and anxious because they are facing their secondary school entrance exams. Their parents push them more and more; they want them to enter better schools.

'My students are lagging three years behind in knowledge. The gap between the children from lower-income families and more privileged families is huge now; richer parents have more resources to help their kids catch up. On the positive side, many local teachers are very rigid about learning new things and new trends, but the pandemic pushed us to embrace online learning and e-tools.'

* * *

School closures were a global issue during the pandemic, but students in Hong Kong experienced the greatest disruptions to their schooling. The sudden and unexpected change from a social school environment to remote learning was a shock for both students and teachers, and it had a detrimental impact on the mental health of many.

A study by the NGO Save the Children in September 2020 found that 39 percent of primary and secondary students in Hong Kong may have developed symptoms of mental health disorders. The study attributed this to the double whammy of the social unrest in 2019 and the pandemic. Almost half (46 percent) of the children surveyed said they felt more worried, 23 percent said they felt more sad, and a disturbing 35 percent described their home environment as tense or fearful during the school suspension (Save the Children, 2020).

The impact was particularly hard on very young children who missed out on a proper kindergarten education, playground time, and play dates. These are all environments where social and emotional development and fine motor skills develop naturally. Many of these children struggled when they entered primary school after the pandemic because they weren't adequately prepared for school life. Some students in lower grades were unable to write their names or the numbers 1 to 10 in sequence (Yiu & Zhao, 2023).

As children transition into adolescence, they enter a crucial stage in their social development. During this time, they form friendships with their peers that can provide support during difficult times and help build resilience. Additionally, they develop executive functioning skills that are essential for goal setting, planning, self-control, and maintaining focus. Students in upper primary school who were affected by the pandemic missed out on this critical period, and many struggled to adjust when schools reopened for face-to-face classes.

At the start of the pandemic, many older students were already grappling with the trauma of witnessing the 2019 anti-government protests. The social unrest sparked a wave of emigration, leaving many students feeling depressed and longing for their classmates and relatives who had departed. This was further exacerbated by three years of social distancing and remote learning. The loss of entire school terms and the cancellation of exams were unsettling, and without a support network of peers, many students lacked the resilience that could have helped them navigate these challenging times.

The official figures provided by the Education Bureau showed a 130 percent increase in 12- to 14-year-olds with mental health disorders from 2018 to 2022. The issues ranged from anxiety and depression to obsessive-compulsive disorder, bipolar and oppositional defiant disorders, and eating problems. The increase was even higher in senior grades. In 2023, the bureau logged 776 students taking sub-degree and undergraduate courses with mental health issues, up from fewer than 300 five years earlier (Yiub, 2023). These figures are most likely on the conservative side, as the bureau only recorded students who had been formally assessed by a clinical psychologist.

The rapid shift to online teaching during the pandemic presented many challenges for teachers, from technical issues to difficulties interacting with students. A report by psychologist Dr Judith Blaine, titled 'Teachers' Mental Wellbeing During Ongoing School Closures in Hong Kong', found that 70 percent of teachers surveyed considered leaving the profession and/or Hong Kong because of school closures. Most cited the government's response and policies about COVID-19 as a reason (Blaine, 2022).

Most of those surveyed by Blaine were from international schools, but the report reflected the exhaustion felt by teachers. In 2021, more than 5,000 teachers resigned, and 30,000 students withdrew from Hong Kong schools (Master & Murdoch, 2022).

Parents' mental health also took a hit during the school closures. A survey by the Hong Kong Paediatric Foundation and the Chinese University of Hong Kong in 2022 found that 20 percent of parents didn't know how to handle the situation. Thirty percent of these parents said their monthly household income had fallen. On a scale of 1 to 10, 10 being the most stressed, 20 percent of parents rated their stress level at 9–10. Those highly stressed parents were more likely to have children who experienced more frequent temper tantrums.

The study found that the happiness index of children of parents with higher stress levels dropped 35 percent (Chinese University of Hong Kong [CUHK]), 2022).

Children and adolescents were especially vulnerable to mental distress during the pandemic. School closures didn't just mean a change in the way they learned; it upset the structure and stability of their lives, leading to psychosocial problems and an increase in bad habits. A large-scale study of more than 29,000 Hong Kong families with children aged 2 to 12 years found that during the pandemic, children spent long periods staring at screens, went to bed later, and got inadequate sleep and exercise (Tso et al., 2022).

Alongside the school closures came a raft of regulations, including the mandatory wearing of face masks in public. Most Hong Kongers had been wearing face masks for several months before the government made it compulsory in July 2020. The extended duration of the mask mandate, which was only lifted on March 1, 2023, has left its mark on many children and is most obviously seen in their speech development.

Children learn pronunciation and phonics by watching and imitating the mouth movement of other people, which wasn't possible when everyone was wearing a face mask. Some children also had difficulty hearing their teacher when she was wearing a mask. Figures released by the Department of Health reveal the extent of the issue: The number of children under 12 with newly diagnosed speech problems and language delay increased from 4,300 in 2019 to 5,401 in 2021 (Yiub, 2023).

The prolonged wearing of face masks meant that children grew up without being able to see the expressions of those around them, limiting their ability to read social cues and stunting their social development. Children who misread their peers' expressions risked being shunned.

When the mask mandate was eventually lifted, most Hong Kongers continued to wear masks. Many young children were anxious about taking off their masks: some said they felt safer with them on since it was what they'd been familiar with for most of their lives. Self-conscious pre-teens who had hidden behind masks as a safety blanket were reluctant to take them off in front of their peers and confront their insecurities.

Strategies and Support

For teachers, self-care is crucial. Only when you take care of your own mental well-being can you effectively support your students. Make sure you are getting enough sleep, eating well, and exercising. Stay connected to friends and family and consider forming a peer-support group to help navigate the changes and stay on top of developments. School closures can be disruptive and overwhelming for students. As their teacher, you can help them feel connected by dividing them into small groups for online activities and encouraging them to exchange contact information. Keep in mind that some students may not have a quiet place to work at home or may be facing family issues, so be flexible and let them know you are there to support them.

For students, staying on top of online learning is key. Start by making a list and breaking down large assignments into smaller tasks, and allow yourself to feel satisfaction for your steady progress. Avoid the temptation to check your social media by putting your phone aside. You can have a quick look at your phone as a reward when you have completed a section of work. Incorporate movement into your day by getting up and walking around or doing star jumps every hour. After finishing online school for the day, go for a walk to get some fresh air. Stick to a routine and stay on track to feel calm. If you're having trouble coming up with a structure, ask for help from a parent, teacher, or classmate. Be kind to yourself as you adapt to change.

For parents, it's important to connect with your child and listen to what's going on for them. Try not to jump in with suggestions or solutions too quickly. If you show that you're really listening and not judging, they'll likely open up more. Being present and letting them feel heard can boost their mental health and strengthen your bond. If your child is struggling with lessons, sit down with them and go through the work together. If you're feeling stressed with your own work and family pressures, suggest a time each day when they can come to you for support. Creating a structure early on, making clear times when you can be available for your child and times when you can't, will help to create stability and reduce conflict.

4

The Elderly

Hong Kong was quick to seal its borders and shut down schools and businesses. Public gatherings of more than two people were banned. The social distancing regulations kept COVID-19 at bay, but they took their toll on people's mental health. Elderly people were particularly affected, many of whom were living alone or in care homes. Their lives were disrupted, and social relationships weakened, leading to increased emotional distress.

For the first two years, the city was largely untouched by the virus, and the oldest and most vulnerable residents remained largely unvaccinated. However, the draconian restrictions ultimately failed to keep the virus out of this densely populated city, and as it swept through Hong Kong in early 2022, elderly people accounted for most of the deaths.

***Joanne** (not her real name) worked as an Intensive Care Unit nurse at Princess Margaret Hospital during the 2003 SARS epidemic. Traumatised by that experience, she left nursing to manage residential* *care homes for the elderly. During the COVID-19 pandemic, she oversaw two homes in Hung Hom and Sai Ying Pun.*

'My daughter was only two years old during the SARS outbreak. I lived away from home because I didn't want to risk infecting my family. Many of the staff were afraid of the disease and resigned. Usually an ICU nurse is in charge of one patient, but we were short-staffed and each of us had to take care of four or five patients. We were working 10 or 11 hours a day. Every night, my husband drove my daughter to the hospital. They stayed in the car with the windows closed so that I could see her for a while. She was too young to understand what was happening.

'During SARS many cases passed away in front of me; it was terrible. Some of my friends and colleagues passed away. Some doctor and nurse friends who I worked with during the day were admitted to ICU in the night and passed away. When I was off duty, I cried a lot. It was really traumatising, and management didn't give us any support. One day the top management came to tell us we'd done well and encouraged us to share our experience. I shared my experience, but when my emotions came, who cared? It made me really angry.

'Two years after SARS, I resigned from my post at the hospital. I told myself it was enough. I had to leave. When COVID started, all those memories of SARS came back. Even though years have passed, I still have many emotions from that time.

'At the beginning of COVID, a few of our elders were sent to a quarantine centre. When they were discharged, they had each lost 15 pounds in body weight. One even lost 20 pounds. The medication we had packed for them was untouched. We said to the staff at the centre, "Did you feed our elders? Did you give them their medication?" But they said, "No comment." Some of the seniors were put in restraints. Even though they could walk, they didn't let them out of bed. They said they didn't want any elders to fall, so they didn't allow them to walk. It was abuse. Some elders told us when they got back that they didn't bathe them, and if they fed them, it was just one or two spoonfuls. If they didn't eat, they were just left. It was heartbreaking to see them come out of quarantine after a few weeks so thin and weak.

'We urged the government and the Social Welfare Department to urge the doctors to come to the care homes and vaccinate our elderly. They said they didn't have the resources and to wait. And then COVID came. Many homes were infected at the end of 2021. Internally, we set up a contingency plan and had an emergency support team. We had everything ready and were waiting for the government to give us more information about infected cases being moved to a quarantine centre. We only had seven single rooms, and I set these aside for isolation use.

'In mid-February 2022, we had an outbreak in the Hung Hom elderly home. My boss arranged a place for me to stay above the care home so I wouldn't risk infecting my family. I stayed there for six weeks. The partitions in the care homes were just 1.6 metres high, which meant the air could circulate and the virus spread easily. Residential care homes are not suitable places for isolation. There were 51 residents in the home. We expected the COVID-positive residents would be moved to a quarantine centre, but they left all the cases at the elderly home. That's why the outbreak was so severe. Every day I spent hours calling different departments, but no one could give me any advice. They just asked me to wait. I felt really lost. The infected cases increased quickly from 5 to 10 and then many more. In the end, more than 90 percent of residents were infected.

'I called the Social Welfare Department. They said, "That's not our responsibility; you'd better call the Centre for Health Protection or the Department of Health." Each department passed it to another. No one shouldered responsibility. There was no plan at all. I still can't find a comprehensive plan or any protocols.

'Then there was an outbreak in our Sai Ying Pun home, but still they didn't transfer any cases to the quarantine centre. I was furious. I said, "You can see the outbreak is severe; why don't you deal with it?" They kept saying, "Why don't you handle it?" When cases became critical, we sent them to hospital. When the hospital discharged them, they didn't do any blood tests or check the Ct value to see if the case was safe to discharge. They discharged residents who were still positive, and that triggered another outbreak. Everything was out of control. The government didn't have any guidelines to tell us how to manage it. We were left to manage it by ourselves.

'One of our residents was 63 and very mobile and social. She enjoyed all the activities at the care home. She got COVID and passed away the next day. She'd had her first vaccination only the day before. Most of the residents had only had one vaccination. The woman who had the bed next to hers cried. She said, "Only yesterday she was alive. Why has she passed away so quickly?"

'I worked many hours a day. I was so tired. At night, the staff called me if a resident was short of breath. Residential care homes only have two oxygen cylinders, but the oxygen levels of many elders were falling. Why were residential homes made into quarantine centres? They weren't equipped for it.

'One day a staff member cried and cried as she told me another elder had died. She asked if there was anything we could do. I asked all the staff to gather. I put on a music CD and talked to them. I am Catholic and wanted to pray for the elders. The staff were all crying. I wanted to give them the chance to express their emotions. I told myself, "Don't fall down; you must keep going or they will feel lost."

I think my religion helped me a lot. Prayer and the support of my family were really important. My daughter met me outside the home and brought food. My boss even offered to come in the home to help, but I told her not to because the outbreak was so severe. She brought me vitamins. That psychological support was very important.

'One by one the elders passed away. In total, eight residents in the Hung Hom care home died. There were COVID deaths in our Sai Ying Pun care home as well. The superintendent of that home felt very guilty and blamed herself. She said to me, "If I could have done more, maybe the elders wouldn't have died." I told her it wasn't her fault and she cried and cried. During the pandemic, everyone was busy dealing with the virus, but no one cared about psychological issues. Even now that the pandemic has passed, still no mental health professional has come.

'I think about all those elders waiting outside the A&E. How could that happen in Hong Kong? The government needs to think about that. But the pandemic has passed, and no one wants to think about it. There is complete silence on this. The government should shoulder its responsibility and formulate guidelines and workflows, particularly for elder homes like ours. The Social Welfare Department has to lead us and give us advice during a pandemic. We need a dedicated hotline for residential care homes that we can call if an elder gets the virus. That only came at the end stage of the pandemic. We want comprehensive protocols for the future. If we have just a wait-and-see approach, when another pandemic comes the same thing may happen.'

Mr Wong *(not his real name), a 76-year-old divorcé, lives by himself in North Point. His son applied for a British National (Overseas) visa* *and moved to the UK with his family two years ago. His daughter still lives in Hong Kong.*

'I never thought I was an emotional person. I am always very steady, but these few years I've been very anxious. In the beginning, I thought it would be like SARS and would go away in a few months. But it didn't. I thought I should be rational and educate myself about the virus. I spent a lot of time on my mobile phone, reading the news, and that really affected my emotions. When I heard about so many people dying around the world and then in Hong Kong, sometimes I couldn't sleep.

'I used to like playing chess with my friends in the park, but when COVID came, my daughter told me not to; she said it was dangerous. Even if I wanted to play chess I couldn't because there was no one there; everyone was staying at home. In the beginning, I walked around the neighbourhood in the morning. It was so troublesome because I had to remember to wear a mask and a face shield. I had to carry a tissue to press the lift button. Germs, germs, I'm always thinking about the germs. And then when I got outside there was not much to do; so many things were closed. In the end, there was not much to do but to stay at home. Why bother getting dressed when you are just going to lie on the bed all day? I was not so quiet before, but I am now. Even when the phone rings sometimes I don't feel like answering it. Too much time by yourself is not a good thing.

'My daughter lives quite close by with her husband and son. Sometimes they visit and bring food, but the mood is not so good because their business is not going too well. Many of her customers have left Hong Kong, and the economy is not very good. She works with her husband, so both of them are struggling, and that makes me worried. It seems like I am worried all the time now; I never used to be like this.

'Now the pandemic is over, but my mood is not like before. Sometimes I meet a friend to play chess in the park, but I don't know what happened to the others. Maybe some of them died? Some of them I don't know their numbers; we just met in the park and became friends. In the summer, my son will bring my granddaughters to Hong Kong. For more than three years I only saw them online. Finally, after so long, I will see them.'

***Uncle Wong**, who is in his 70s, is retired and lives in a small room in a subdivided flat in Tai Kok Tsui. The flat is on the third floor of a tenement building that has no lift. Despite walking with a noticeable limp, Uncle Wong says he had grown accustomed to the climb.*

'I remember SARS 20 years ago. That was quite short; it lasted just a few months, but the COVID pandemic was different—it went on for three years and was a lot more serious. So many more people died from COVID than from SARS. I never expected to experience something like that in my life. It really affected me and changed the way I think about life. Now I try to appreciate every day and live for the moment. Whatever is happening around us, we still need to live, so why spend time getting worried? Maybe it is the wisdom of being older.

'During the pandemic, Hong Kong was like a dead city; the streets were so quiet and there were hardly any people in the restaurants. I took the opportunity to travel around Hong Kong. I went to the New Territories and around Hong Kong Island. Now that the city is busy again, I stay mostly in Tai Kok Tsui.

'I got my information about COVID from the TV news and the newspaper. Some of the news was very dramatic, and there were frightening stories about the vaccine and what might happen if you took the vaccine. It was mainly those stories that made me decide to wait until the last minute to get vaccinated. I treated COVID like a normal flu or cold. The way I saw it, there was nothing I could do; I still had to live. I didn't want to rely on the vaccine. I think my body is quite strong. If I had a choice, I wouldn't have got vaccinated. I only did it when the government made it compulsory to have the vaccine if you wanted to go into a restaurant.

'I've been retired for more than 10 years. Most of that time I've been living in an 80-square-foot room in a subdivided flat. The flat is divided into five small rooms, and eight of us live there and we share the toilet and the kitchen. A couple live in one room with their son. The mother got COVID first, then her husband and then the son. They stayed in their room, but they still had to use the shared toilet; there was no choice. I didn't get COVID.

'I went to the ImpactHK community centre in Tai Kok Tsui. It was open through the pandemic, and there is air-con and a computer, so it is easy to spend my time there. I have met a lot of friends there. I'm not in contact with my family, and the people I've met at ImpactHK feel like family.

'The COVID policies changed every day and people had to keep adapting, which was very stressful for the community. If we have another pandemic, I hope that we learn from the experience of COVID-19 and it won't be as bad.

'So many people died during COVID, especially the elderly. It made me feel that life is unpredictable; you just have to let it be. Before the pandemic I didn't have this attitude, but the pandemic made me realise that there are a lot of things that you can't control. Everything is down to fate. I've learned to go with the flow.'

* * *

In 2022, more than one-fifth of the city's population, or 20.8 percent of its 7.48 million people, were aged over 65. This group is expected to increase to 25.3 percent by 2028. And increasingly they are living alone. According to government census figures, the number of elderly people living by themselves rose by more than 50 percent from 2006 to 2016. This population is particularly vulnerable during a pandemic in both their physical and mental health.

In February 2020, the scramble for face masks amid the shortage of protective gear worried many. This was particularly concerning for the elderly population, who are more susceptible to the virus and its complications. The emotional distress experienced by this group was evident early on in the pandemic.

'Many of the city's elderly couldn't obtain masks and became extremely anxious. Some even thought they were going to die, they were that scared,' said Maura Wong Hung-hung, CEO of Senior Citizen Home Safety Association in an interview with the *South China Morning Post* (Wong, 2020).

Then came the isolation caused by the social-distancing measures. The closure of the centres for the elderly, public libraries, and swimming pools brought a halt to their social life and upended daily routines. Restaurants only allowed tables for two people and closed at 6 pm. No more than two families could gather in private premises, and no visitors were allowed in elderly care homes. In addition, many at-home services for the elderly, such as meal deliveries, were cancelled. All this chipped away at their social support and heightened their sense of isolation.

As the city shut down, people turned to their smartphones to keep abreast of the fast-changing news and stay in touch with friends and family. A survey found that only 28 percent of people aged 80 and above used a smartphone, further aggravating their social isolation (CUHK, 2021).

Staying at home and avoiding social interactions were strategies intended to keep elderly people, an at-risk group, physically safe. But it meant they meant they no longer received the social and emotional support they had previously gained from social interactions and activities. As humans, we need social connection to help us regulate our emotions and cope with stress. Loneliness and social isolation compound feelings of stress, which has a negative impact on our physical and mental health.

As the weeks dragged on, that isolation turned to depression. In July 2021, the suicide prevention group Samaritan Befrienders Hong Kong recorded 446 deaths by suicide of people older than 60, the highest yearly number since 1973 (The Samaritan Befrienders Hong Kong [SBHK]), 2022).

Many seniors were reluctant to get vaccinated against COVID-19. The early success in containing the virus led to complacency—the sense that COVID-19 was a menace elsewhere in the world but that Hong Kong was safe. This complacency was compounded by baseless fears that older people and those in poor health were especially at risk from vaccines. As a result, many people believed that if border controls and social distancing measures were effective, vaccination was not a priority.

In June 2021, only five percent of 70- to 79-year-olds were vaccinated, and just one percent of those over 80 had been jabbed. The Hong Kong College of Physicians appealed for the staff and residents at old age homes to get vaccinated for their physical as well as mental health. Increased protection, they reasoned, would allow the residential homes to increase visiting hours and allow elderly residents to go out, which would boost their mood and resilience (Li, 2021).

But the vaccine uptake remained low. It wasn't until COVID-19 began spreading quickly through the city in early 2022 that there was a rush to get vaccinated. By the end of March 2022, 80 percent of 70- to 79-year-olds had at least one dose of the vaccine, and 57 percent of 80-year-olds (Hong Kong Baptist University [HKBU]), 2022).

By then many elderly residents had spent two years in isolation, either in cramped flats or in care homes, where they were cut off from their families. Emotions ran high, fluctuating between anxiety, sadness, and anger. With the news of the high fatality rate among unvaccinated older people, many felt both hopeless and helpless. Many older adults didn't know how or where to look for help. A study of almost 5,000 seniors during the deadly fifth wave found that more than one-third were suffering from emotional distress. Many (29 percent) were experiencing loneliness, 14 percent showed signs of depression, and 12 percent were anxious. Their greatest COVID-related concern was being a burden to their family if they were infected with the virus (University of Hong Kong, 2022b).

The healthcare system was overwhelmed, and images of elderly people left waiting for days outside hospitals on ambulance gurneys were splashed across front pages and on social media. In March 2022, 15 people over the age of 61 committed suicide in one week. Three of those people had recently tested positive for COVID-19.

Many of Hong Kong's 796 care homes are in the city. Their highly dense structure aided the rapid transmission of the virus. On February 22, 2022, 40 care homes were infected with COVID-19, and two weeks later that number had leapt to 755 (Das, 2022). The majority (90 percent) of care homes used partitions to separate bed spaces, giving residents a degree of privacy while allowing daylight to reach the rooms in the interior of the facility. This design proved lethal in the pandemic, as it allowed for easy transmission of the airborne virus, making the care homes disaster zones.

Many care homes staff resigned out of fear of contracting the virus and bringing it back to their own families. Those who stayed locked themselves in and did their best to look after their elderly residents. The public healthcare system was overwhelmed, quarantine camps were full, and care homes were asked to look after their residents. Staff were distraught as they tried to manage the outbreak in facilities which were not designed to quarantine people. Many engaged empathically with their elderly charges and went on to experience vicarious trauma or secondary traumatic stress.

During the peak of the pandemic in February to May 2022, more than 9,000 people died, and over 5,000 of them were unvaccinated elderly people who were mostly in elderly care homes.

The government has called for an overhaul of care homes, most of which are privately run, in the wake of the pandemic, new design regulations to be phased in. However, the poor mental health of the staff and surviving residents of the care homes where COVID-19 ran amok has yet to be addressed.

Strategies and Support

Even before COVID-19, the health needs of many older people were lacking, as evidenced by the high suicide rate. The pandemic has only made things worse. The key challenge is identifying and treating mental health issues early on, before they become more serious. This can be especially difficult for seniors, who often don't know how to ask for help or are afraid of being a burden.

The community has a role to play in addressing the issue. Family members, friends, and neighbours can help by keeping an eye out for senior people and taking the time to listen to them. This can help reduce their sense of isolation and provide an opportunity to flag any urgent needs that may arise. Seniors can then be connected with the appropriate social services. Family members can provide care and encouragement to help seniors rebuild their lives and introduce meaningful activities into their daily routines.

During the pandemic, social distancing regulations had a disproportionate impact on seniors, who relied on social contact outside of their homes. The heavy reliance on technology and smartphones to stay connected and navigate the rapidly changing regulations further isolated many seniors. Supporting elderly people with technology can help relieve their anxiety and make them feel more included.

Seniors must be involved in decisions about their own mental health and have a choice about how they receive support. However, often they need gentle support and guidance to help them understand their options and feel less isolated. Communication and connectedness are key.

Older adults are a diverse group with varying physical and mental capacities that extend beyond their chronological age. Some may choose to volunteer to support their peers by teaming up with social workers to call on other older adults, understand their needs, and offer companionship to reduce loneliness. By being actively engaged in supporting others, they gain a sense of purpose and bolster their resilience.

Even after the pandemic, many older people still feel isolated. It's common for them to lose connections within their social network and find it hard to start new friendships. We need not wait until the next pandemic to help these people feel more socially connected.

5

Pandemic Pregnancy

In an open letter to Hong Kong's leading English-language newspaper, three expectant mothers expressed their apprehensions about the predicament that pregnant women were facing amidst the pandemic. Their voices echoed the concerns of many, highlighting the challenges and uncertainties that came with bringing new life into the world during such unprecedented times.

'Giving birth should be a moment of the most joyful anticipation for parents-to-be, not apprehension. Yet, we live in fear of what this moment will bring,' wrote Florence Sai Wing Chan, Puja Kapai, and Victoria Wisniewski Otero in the *South China Morning Post* (Chan, 2022).

In their March 2022 letter, the women highlighted three primary concerns: the ambiguity about parent-child separation policies; the prohibition of birth partners in delivery rooms at public hospitals; and the refusal of private hospitals to admit COVID-positive women in labour. They also expressed uncertainty about how expectant mothers and their partners should prepare for admission to public hospitals and what to expect if they or their newborns tested positive for COVID-19. This uncertainty was further exacerbated by the constantly changing landscape as certain public hospitals were designated for COVID-19 patient care and there were conflicting reports on how similar cases were being handled.

The women concluded their letter with a plea for the implementation of humane, clear, and science-based protocols that prioritise holistic child and maternal care while also adhering to necessary health and safety measures. They emphasised the importance of effectively communicating these protocols to both frontline staff and the public to ensure that everyone is well-informed and prepared.

Monique*, a first-time mother, found it challenging trying to keep up with the ever-changing COVID-19 regulations. She gave birth in February 2022, during the height of Hong Kong's pandemic. Shortly after delivery, her baby was taken away without any explanation, leaving Monique traumatised and desperate to be reunited with her newborn.*

'The lead-up to the birth was very stressful because the regulations were changing constantly, and even the hospital staff didn't know what the protocols were. The hospital wasn't accepting anyone who tested positive or was a close contact. We knew we needed a negative PCR test to be allowed into the hospital. So, every couple of days for three weeks leading up to my due date we submitted PCR tests at a community centre, to make sure we had a valid result.

'There were a lot of horror stories going around about what happened if you tested positive. One was that there was an unofficial maternity ward in the basement of an isolation facility where they would take you. I don't know if that was true, but the stories that my pregnant friends and I were hearing were scary.

'I prepared as best I could. I made a playlist to distract me from the contractions, and my bag was packed and ready with snacks and my phone. The week she was due, the government started issuing lots of compulsory testing notices. Suddenly, it was taking five days to get the PCR test results back.

'My waters broke at 1 am, and our most recent result was outside the 48-hour window. We went to Prince of Wales Hospital, and they let me in to do a COVID test. I was a long way off giving birth, but because it was taking seven hours to get the results back from the lab, they were telling women to come in as soon as their waters broke. After I'd done the test, I asked to see my husband and was told, "It's not allowed. He's gone home."

'Ideally, I would have been getting some rest ahead of the birth, but I was in a ward with people who were having contractions and screaming in agony. I got contractions at about 8 am and was moved to the early labour ward. I thought my bag would move with me, but it didn't. They said I would get it in the post-delivery ward. That rattled me. I wanted my phone to call my husband. I wanted my things. I wanted to stand up and stretch my legs and let gravity play its part, but they wouldn't let me stand even within the curtained-off area around my bed. They wouldn't even let me have my feet on the floor. Every time I asked why I couldn't do something they said, "It's because of COVID."

'I was thirsty but they wouldn't let me drink. They wouldn't let me eat. I wasn't even allowed to go to the bathroom, and they kept putting a bedpan under me. I was told there was a ward phone that was shared, but each time I asked, they said someone was using it. I don't know if it existed, or COVID meant we weren't allowed to share a ward phone.

'Everyone tells you to try and stay Zen and focus on your breathing, but I was thinking, "Where is my stuff? I can't move from my bed. I can't speak to my husband." The midwives were worried because I was only 1 cm dilated. I said, "I'm not very relaxed right now. I just want to talk to my husband. I want my stuff." Logic was out of the window.

'When I was eventually moved to the delivery ward, there was a different set of nurses. They let me have little sips of water. I was upset that I couldn't speak to my husband and keep him posted. Somehow, we got a message to him that he should come. When he arrived, my whole demeanour changed. I could finally relax and focus and tell him what happened. He held my hand and helped me get through the contractions. Having him there helped so much. Two and a half hours after he arrived, I was pushing and had fully dilated after so many hours of not going past 1 cm.

'Suddenly, alarms started going off, lights started pinging, and my husband was thrown out of the room. Paperwork was thrust in front of me to sign. What was happening? I had no idea what I was signing. It turned out that because I had dilated so quickly, I had to have my baby suctioned out. Up until then I'd only been dealing with midwives, but suddenly a doctor rushed in with 10 students. He said, "Your baby is in extreme distress; relax and push when I say."

'The next thing I know, I have my baby in my arms. She was fine, I was fine, and they were stitching me up. I asked where my husband was and they said, "He's gone home." I said, "Has anyone told him I'm ok, that the baby is ok?" My baby had just been born and here I was arguing.

'Immediately after I'd given birth, they took my temperature. It was 37.5 degrees. They took it again 15 minutes later and it was back to normal. This I only found out later.

'I went to the post-delivery ward, where I was reunited with my things and my phone. I was with my baby and everything was fine. At 11 pm, a nurse appeared and took my baby from me. She didn't say why; she just took her. I asked what she was doing, and she said, "The baby is at risk of developing something because you had an elevated temperature. I am taking her to the special care baby unit."

'I was upset. I said I felt fine and asked her not to do anything to my baby without asking me first. I thought she'd bring her back in an hour or so, but she didn't. I was awake all night. In the morning I was in pieces and asked the nurse what was happening to my baby. She said, "Client confidentiality. We can't tell you anything."

'Later that day, I spoke to a doctor. He said the nurse meant to say that the postnatal ward didn't have access to the special care baby unit, which is why she didn't have information to share with me. I was told my baby had been given antibiotics, put on a drip, and had X-rays done.

"What's wrong with her?" I asked.

"We are running tests."

I was angry and upset. I was alone and in pieces. Beyond the curtain, I could hear babies all around me. A nurse saw me crying and asked what was wrong.

"I've just given birth and my baby has been taken away," I said.

But she just didn't get it.

'I discharged myself and went to the special care baby unit and camped out with my husband. Eventually a doctor came out. Making sure to speak calmly and rationally, I told him that I didn't want to overstep anything, but I wanted to go through the tests.

'I reassured him, "If there's any indication she needs to be there, then of course she must stay. But if there's no need for her to be kept there, then I think it's better she's with her mum getting skin on skin and breast milk."

'That was when I learned that my temperature immediately after giving birth was 37.5 degrees, which is considered an elevated temperature. I also learned my temperature had returned to normal when it was checked 15 minutes later. That brief elevated temperature was the reason why they'd taken her away.

'I went through all the test results with the doctor. Everything was in the normal range; there was nothing unusual. I think the doctor appreciated that I wasn't being reckless and emotional. He eventually got the lawyers at the hospital to prepare papers to say we were discharging against medical advice. That was a petrifying thing to do as a new parent, but I was so sure she needed to be home with her mum.

'It was not a nice way to start the journey of parenthood.

'I'm in a mums' group of 10 women. We all had our babies within two weeks of each other. Seven of us in the group had our babies taken to the special care baby unit or neonatal intensive care unit immediately after birth. All the babies were put on antibiotics and given X-rays. I was the only one who discharged against medical advice, and the others didn't get their babies back for four or more days.

'I understand that there was a lot of caution because of the pandemic, but the bedside manner could have been better. If the nurse who took my baby away had explained what was happening, it would have been a lot less stressful. If I'd been kept informed about what was happening, that would have been reassuring.

'One of the hardest things about being pregnant during the pandemic was that no one really knew what was happening. The uncertainty could have been better managed if there was one place where the current regulations and information was posted so that everyone—parents, doctors, and nurses—could be on the same page and informed. If the regulations change every hour, then it can be changed on a very public notice area so that everyone is clear.'

At the start of the pandemic, ***Samantha*** *(not her real name) discovered that she was expecting her first child. Concerned about stories circulating of women being separated from their newborns in public hospitals, she and her husband made the decision to save up for a private hospital.*

'We'd been trying for quite a long time have a baby. I got pregnant in February 2020 and in March went to Australia for a short trip. When I got to Australia, people were really nervous when they heard that I'd come from Hong Kong, and so China, because this new virus was seen as a Chinese infection.

'As my pregnancy progressed, it became apparent the pandemic wasn't going to go away, and Hong Kong's approach was going to be quite authoritarian and risk-averse. In some ways that was assuring, but in other ways it made me nervous about what it would mean for my pregnancy and the birth.

'As a pregnant woman, I found wearing a mask through the summer very uncomfortable. In the heat, the face covering was claustrophobic and horrible. I'd be sucking the mask to my face because I was trying to breathe. One morning, during my first trimester, I had morning sickness in a taxi on the way to work and vomited into my mask.

'Pregnancy is a time when things are unpredictable. Not being able to do the things that might have made me feel good was upsetting. The swimming pools were closed; things were shutting down. Because the restrictions were changing all the time, there were lots of made and cancelled plans. In the late stage of pregnancy, it wasn't ideal.

'Public hospitals are usually very good and safe in Hong Kong, but during the pandemic it became apparent that they would require you to keep your mask on through the birth, that your partner couldn't be there with you, and if you tested positive there was a high chance that they would take your baby away. My husband and I decided to go private. It was a decision that upset me. I'm not someone normally driven by fear, but I was feeling quite vulnerable. I was in very privileged position that I could do that. We saved to do it, and I wouldn't have done it if not for the pandemic.

'I decided to have an induction. This was partly medical, but also so that a date could be set for the birth. My husband and I locked down and worked from home for two weeks so we could reduce our risk of getting COVID. From 38 and a half weeks, I was doing a PCR test every three days to make sure I had a negative test on hand. If I'd tested positive, I wouldn't have been allowed into the private hospital. I would have gone into the public system, and there were lots of stories of babies being taken away.

'In the summer of 2021, we took our baby on holiday to meet her grandparents. On the way there, we were very excited about spending time with people we cared about. Travel was difficult. While we were away, our flights got cancelled twice and we had to shift country. At the end of a long journey back, we had to spend three weeks in a quarantine hotel. My husband and I were both vaccinated, so we only needed to do a week of quarantine, but because our nine-month-old hadn't been vaccinated, we had to do three weeks.

'A few days into our quarantine, the rules changed, and quarantine time was reduced, but they wouldn't let us out. We had friends with children who were going into quarantine after us and getting out before us. We were pretty devastated. We tried to make the best of it as much as possible. On the positive side, we noticed the baby coming on in leaps and bounds. But there were real moments of anger and frustration at the rules which didn't seem to make sense. What was the point of keeping us locked up when the quarantine rules had changed?

'My second pregnancy was harder, probably because I now had a toddler. The baby classes and things like that which I would have taken her to weren't on. She was in the house a lot more than we would have hoped and wasn't running off steam.

'One of the first words my little girl said was "mask", which was quite depressing. She was keen to wear a mask, which was also quite sad. We were worried about the mask affecting her speech development. When I was seven months pregnant, there was a policy that if you tested positive you could isolate at home unless you were considered an "at-risk person", which meant unvaccinated individuals (children under two), or you were pregnant. It would have meant we'd either have to leave our daughter at home or bring her to Penny's Bay. It was fear inducing. I understand the macro, but it did drive fear, which is something I don't usually associate with protocols and policies.

'Towards the end of my second pregnancy, I couldn't believe we were in the same situation. It felt galling and stressful that it was happening again. The fifth wave was peaking, and it was quite possible that I'd test positive, and I was thinking a lot about what to do to manage my job and keep the baby safe while feeling physically fragile myself. We elected to have the baby induced at 38 and a half weeks. It felt like well within the safe zone; he'd be very much cooked and ready to go. It was safer than waiting until further into the pregnancy, and if I'd tested positive then, there was every chance it wouldn't come for a week.

'It was even more frustrating the second time around. Here I was having to make a similar decision because of similar principles I didn't agree with on how mums and babies should be treated. It was a decision driven by fear rather than by choice. Our second child had some abnormal test results and had to go to Children's Hospital. We were worried that he would be admitted as an in-patient. It felt like additional layers of stuff that you shouldn't need to worry about.

'When I look back on that time, I see that everyone was scared of the virus because of the way people were interacting with it. There was so much fear: It would have been better to treat COVID as an illness that someone is sick with rather than something to be scared of.'

* * *

Pregnancy is already a stressful time, but the pandemic introduced a whole new set of challenges for expectant mothers. They were forced to navigate a world where antenatal exercise classes, seminars, hospital tours, and postnatal classes were all suspended. Visits to mothers and babies staying in postnatal wards were not permitted. Due to the conflicting and ever-changing health advice, including questions about the advisability of getting vaccinated or receiving a booster shot, tensions were high. The lack of information and the spread of fake news only served to exacerbate the stress.

High levels of stress and anxiety experienced by expectant mothers can have potential negative impacts on both the mother and child. Research has shown that women who experience depression, anxiety, and high levels of stress during pregnancy are at an increased risk of perinatal complications and problems later on

(Fransson et al., 2011). These issues can also affect the child; studies link high levels of maternal stress during pregnancy to emotional and behavioural problems in children (Van den Bergh et al., 2005).

The anxiety felt by expectant mothers during the pandemic is not just anecdotal. A study conducted by United Christian Hospital in Hong Kong surveyed 623 women and found that the vast majority—83.1 percent—were worried about contracting COVID-19 during their pregnancy. A similar number, 87 percent, reported only leaving their homes when necessary during the pandemic. And 71.3 percent of the women surveyed expressed concern about getting COVID-19 during their antenatal visits to public hospitals. In fact, 28.9 percent of those women reported bringing their own disinfectant to clean the chair and the examination bed at the clinic before their consultation (Lok et al., 2022).

In that same study, more than 80 percent of the women objected to banning their husbands from accompanying them during labour and delivery. In a pre-pandemic world, the Hospital Authority allowed at least one companion—be it a partner, family member, or friend—to be present in the delivery room. This continuous companion support during labour has been advocated for years in obstetric units across all Hong Kong public hospitals. However, on January 26, 2020, this rule was abruptly suspended, when the first wave of coronavirus hit Hong Kong. Tragically, this measure was not publicly announced, leaving some couples to discover it only after being admitted to the maternity ward.

According to the World Health Organization's (WHO) 2022 guidelines, all pregnant women and their newborns—including those who are COVID-19 positive—have a right to high-quality medical care. The WHO recommends that all women have a companion of choice available throughout labour. This recommendation is backed by a Cochrane review, which found that having a companion for support during labour reduced the rate of caesarean section, duration of labour, instrumental vaginal delivery, need for pain relief, and negative feelings about childbirth experiences (Bohren et al., 2017). Additionally, women without the support of a partner are more likely to have babies who struggle with immediate breastfeeding (Fan et al., 2022).

Joanne Li's experience highlights the difficulties of giving birth without the support of a partner. In 2019, when she had her first child, her husband was by her side throughout the labour, cradling her head and urging her to push. However, when she gave birth at a public hospital in February 2022, he was not allowed to enter the hospital.

'This time it was so different because I was alone. It was more painful, and I kept thinking, "I cannot do it." I almost wanted to give up,' she told the *South China Morning Post* (Westbrook, 2022).

While the most contentious issue for new mothers was the barring of partners from delivery rooms, the suspension of visiting hours for mothers and newborns came a close second. A 2020 study of 733 new mothers in Hong Kong found that more than 80 percent considered visits to be a crucial part of their overall pregnancy experience. This was particularly true for Chinese mothers, who made up 85 percent of the study. The traditional Chinese postpartum practice known as 'doing the month' involves new mothers following a specific set of rules for a month after delivery. During this time, the new mother is expected to spend most of the month convalescing in bed and receiving nutritious supplements. However, the suspension of visiting hours meant they were unable to receive that support from close family members (Hui et al., 2022).

In July 2020, Hong Kong saw its first case of a COVID-19-positive mother giving birth. She delivered via emergency caesarean section and the baby was immediately separated from her. During the pandemic, separating newborns from COVID-19 positive mothers or those suspected of being COVID positive was standard practice in Hong Kong.

The COVID-19 pandemic brought with it a wave of fear and uncertainty; and for some women who gave birth during this turbulent time, the impact was profound and will have long-lasting effects on them and their child. A study conducted by researchers at the University of Hong Kong's School of Nursing surveyed 3,027 pregnant and new mothers in Hong Kong and mainland China during the pandemic. The results were alarming: Half of the women reported feeling scared and nervous when thinking about the virus, and a staggering 20 percent suffered postpartum depression, compared with an average 14 percent pre-pandemic. The study found a clear correlation between the women with a high-level of fear of COVID-19 and those who experienced depression (Fan et al., 2022).

However, there was a silver lining to the study: It found that the more knowledge women had about how to prevent COVID-19 infection, the less fearful they were of the virus. This suggests that providing expectant mothers with accurate information about how to protect themselves and their babies could be a key strategy in mitigating the negative impact of future pandemics.

Strategies and Support / Self-Compassion

Self-compassion is all about being kind to yourself, recognising that your experiences are part of what makes us all human, and staying mindful even when times are tough. It can be a powerful tool for new mothers: It's been shown to help protect against postnatal depression. By practising self-compassion, women can better cope with the emotional ups and downs of the perinatal period and reduce their risk of developing mental illness (Muramoto et al., 2022).

We often treat ourselves with far less kindness and compassion than we show to the people we care about. Self-compassion is all about turning that around and including ourselves in our own circle of compassion. It means treating yourself with the same care and kindness that you would show to a good friend who's going through a tough time.

Practising self-compassion starts with acknowledging and validating our own pain instead of trying to ignore or suppress it. It's important to maintain a balanced point of view and not exaggerate the situation. A key aspect of self-compassion is recognising that suffering is something we all share. When we remember that everyone has their own struggles and imperfections, we can feel less alone and more connected to others. And finally, try talking to yourself with a warm and compassionate tone, saying the words you need to hear to comfort or reassure yourself: 'I'm so sorry you're struggling' or 'It's going to be okay'.

Research has shown that people who practise self-compassion are less likely to struggle with anxiety, depression, and stress. And it's not that they're good at ignoring negative experiences—quite the opposite, in fact. With a self-compassionate approach, instead of trying to push away painful feelings and replace them with 'better' ones, we can generate positive emotions by embracing our suffering with kindness and care. This allows us to experience both light and dark at the same time, and this kind and caring attitude can help us better cope with difficulties and find the silver linings in tough situations.

Exercise 1: How Would You Treat a Friend?

1. Consider a situation where a close friend is feeling down or facing a difficult challenge. How do you react to your friend in these circumstances (when you are at your best)? Please record your typical actions and words, as well as the tone of your voice when speaking to your friend.
2. Now, reflect on moments when you are feeling low or facing a struggle. How do you usually react to yourself in these situations? Please record your typical actions and words, as well as the tone of your voice when speaking to yourself.
3. Did you observe any differences? If yes, ask yourself why. What factors or fears influence you to treat yourself and others differently?
4. Record how you think things might change if you reacted to your own suffering in the same way you typically react to a close friend.
5. The next time you face a challenge, try treating yourself like a good friend and observe what happens.

Exercise 2: Self-Compassion Break

This is a way to help you remember to apply the three core components of self-compassion—mindfulness, common humanity, and kindness—when facing difficulties in life. Start by thinking of a situation that is causing you stress. As you bring it to mind, pay attention to where you feel the tension and emotional discomfort in your body.

1. Say to yourself: 'This is a moment of struggle'. You might prefer to say 'This hurts' or 'This is stressful'. The important thing is to acknowledge that you are experiencing difficulty.

2. Next, say to yourself: 'Struggle is a part of life'. You could also say 'Lots of people struggle just like this' or 'I'm not alone'. In this way, you can connect with others who also experience similar struggles. You may want to put your hands over your heart and feel the warmth of your hands on your chest.
3. Finally, say: 'May I be kind to myself'. If that doesn't feel right, you could say 'May I learn to accept myself as I am' or 'May I be patient with myself'.

Keep in mind that self-compassion isn't about avoiding uncomfortable emotions. It involves mindfully acknowledging that the moment is painful, treating ourselves with kindness, and recognising that imperfection is a common part of the human experience.

6

Frontline Health Workers

Frontline healthcare workers are known for being resilient and trained to deal with illness and death. However, even before the pandemic, their mental health and psychological well-being was identified as a major healthcare issue. With the arrival of COVID-19, healthcare workers were under immense pressure. The manifold stressors—the risk of infection, worries of transmission to family members at home, shortage of personal protective equipment (PPE), long shifts, and heavier workload—made these dedicated workers at risk of anxiety, depression, sleeping disorders, and burnout.

Doctors and nurses put themselves and their loved ones at risk every day to care for their patients. They didn't have the luxury of taking time off or working from home. All the while, they coped with the trauma of witnessing significant loss. The emotional exhaustion that came with the job caused anxiety, depression, and reduced mental well-being (Dinibutun, 2020). It was a feeling of being tired and emotionally worn down that led to a lack of energy and feeling overloaded on the job. These professionals took on the role of looking after others, often without a moment to take care of themselves. Despite the challenges they faced, they found meaning in their work. In conversations with these professionals, they often report strong team cohesiveness and comradery.

***Dr Lam** (not her real name), a paediatrician in her 30s, received her education in both Hong Kong and the United Kingdom. Like many doctors, she suffered from a lack of sleep prior to the pandemic. Following the outbreak of COVID-19, sleep deprivation became chronic and exacerbated her stress.*

'The public system accounts for 90 percent of hospitalisations, but we have only 40 percent of the city's healthcare workers. For decades we've been running with a personnel shortage and resources issue. During the 2019 protests, frontline workers who provided neutral aid for both protesters and police were arrested and accused of collusion. This smear campaign led to a breakdown of trust. We started seeing a massive exodus. People began leaving at the beginning of the pandemic. We lost 4.6 percent of nurses and doctors by 2020, and it's been a steady brain drain since.

'In late 2019, I got back from a year of training in the UK. In early December, I heard reports from friends in Shanghai and other parts of China of an emerging virus. It seemed there was a big viral thing coming and we should be prepared. I was living with my parents. They are getting old and my dad has diabetes. I knew I would be called to the front line, so in January [2020] I moved into a hotel in Sheung Wan because I didn't want to risk infecting them. Hotels were making good offers at the time, so I got a room for HK$10,000 a month.

'At the beginning there was a shortage of PPE. This wasn't new; the healthcare system has long been under-resourced. We were worried about infecting our family members; it was an extra stress.

The PPE was being rationed. Every time you gown up you've used one kit, so if you were dirty you stayed dirty for a 12-hour shift. It was stressful. I was tired and exhausted. There was no end point; it was impossible to plan for anything.

'I was in high school during SARS in 2003, but I had colleagues who had lost family members and colleagues. There was an implicit understanding there was a lot of risk. I was anxious for my parents. There was never an issue of whether I was going to show up. This is a system that relies on the goodwill of its workers. We are all fairly young.

'As the pandemic dragged on, one of the hardest parts for me was the social isolation. We were rostered onto either a dirty—working with COVID patients—or a clean team. As healthcare workers, a lot of our social support is other healthcare workers. However, we were all isolating at work and eating alone. Everything was about infection control; you don't want cross-infection among groups. If one colleague got COVID, we'd all have been in quarantine as close contacts. The sense of camaraderie I'd had with my team was suddenly gone. Outside work, I wasn't seeing my friends. I wasn't seeing anyone. The extent we went to, to protect our families, by not bringing the virus home, was at the expense of our mental health.

'We were already short-staffed, and now we had a critical human resources issue with staff deployed from all over. We were creating human resources out of nothing. A friend who is a dermatologist was put in charge of the COVID camps. People were asking, "Am I competent to manage what I've been assigned to do?" The skills mismatch was a big part of the anxiety at work. Everyone who was redeployed was out of their depth. If you are not in a setting where you are useful, there is guilt.

'I stayed at the hotel in Sheung Wan until the end of April 2020. Every day I went from my hotel room to work and back again. It wasn't a home. I was eating a lot of takeout. I got a hotpot that I could plug in and make a little hotpot for dinner, but that got old fast. It was subsistence living. It was impossible to get days off because we were running the clean and dirty rosters and were banned from travel. My parents were isolating, and I was isolating. I wasn't seeing my social network of healthcare workers; everyone was exhausted. I thought it would be a matter of weeks, and it turned into months and it went on.

'By mid-2020, as the community had higher levels of infection and the precautions became clearer, people became more comfortable about socialising. I moved into a flat 10 minutes from the hospital. It was a place I could put my head down and ease my anxiety. I started batch-cooking for the week ahead. The meal preparation helped me to destress.

'With each wave it was very frustrating because we couldn't plan our services. Every time someone was deployed, we had to redo the schedule. Arrangements for the unexpected waves of COVID were hard to deal with. Healthcare professionals were constantly playing catch-up on recommendations. It was also stressful for GPs. How could they keep up with the recommendations?

'Our hospital wasn't built for the pandemic. Our isolation rooms were designed for one child and one parent. We saw a massive influx of people, so we had to put four cots in one room, which meant there wasn't space to accommodate the adults. We couldn't even squeeze in a chair and had to move the cots to reach each patient. Parents offered to sleep in the corridor, but often they were also COVID positive, so that wasn't possible. Children not having their carer with them is our worst nightmare, but we just didn't have the capacity to house them at the same time. There was a lot of misunderstanding about this issue. Part of it is a cultural problem—I don't think we acknowledged there is a language barrier for people who don't speak Cantonese. There was not enough translation. We were overloading a system that was already overloaded. We were getting requests from parents to read to their child or sing to them every hour. But when you are that busy it is subsistence care—you look after them medically, feed them. All we can do is keep them alive.

'When it came to child separation, there would have been better ways to settle this, but we were running from patient to patient. When you have a breakdown in trust and communication, and it's no one's fault, it's frustrating. I felt quite helpless. We were already doing our best. There were conversations I wanted to have, but I couldn't because I was rushing between patients who were crashing. If a parent doesn't see me, it's probably that I'm looking after a child who is sicker than theirs. We didn't have enough staff. We didn't have time to eat or drink. It was physically impossible for us to sit down and explain the situation to every parent.

'All of this came on top of the existing stress of being public healthcare staff. From the day you qualify, you don't sleep. The lack of sleep is chronic; you are prioritising other people over your own health. You are on call for 36 hours and terrified of missing a call. If you miss a call the patient is screwed, so a lot of us are light sleepers. I worry about my patients, and that keeps me going. I don't think I've slept well, except on annual leave. During the pandemic, I was sleeping three or four hours a night for weeks on end. Then there might be a few quiet weeks, and it would be back to three or four hours. In a high-pressure situation, you are running on adrenaline.

'From a mental health perspective, it's about having the time to destress. All of us have accumulated a lot of annual leave, but we can't take it because we need to clear the backlog of cases. We were already experiencing chronic anxiety, and the pandemic just increased the decibel. Now it's over and we are back to basic levels of anxiety and exhaustion. I don't think we even register it as a problem. I feel numb. I don't think I realise the degree to which my mental health has taken a hit. Many of us in the industry don't think about our own mental health. Whatever you are feeling is superseded by looking after someone else.

'It is an issue of human resources. If we'd had enough people at work on a normal basis, we could have stretched it out and covered it. We should have learned from SARS in 2003 and invested more in increasing the number of student placements. We know we are haemorrhaging people in Hong Kong and not covering the gaps. It is a gradual attrition and we are not doing anything about it.

'This is a high-demand, high-stakes environment where people make errors. We want to move away from a toxic work environment and towards an environment that promotes mental well-being. One where everyone works harder on their days in, and we encourage people to take time off. And when they are away, we try not to call them. There's a hierarchy in hospitals. Elsewhere in the world they are moving towards team collaboration, hearing all voices and encouraging diversity. It's not within Chinese culture to do that; we are inherently hierarchy based. A lot of predominately Chinese staff work cultures would find it difficult to voice different opinions. You might be a young hotshot coming in and wanting to revamp the system, but the system isn't ready.'

Dr Chan *(not his real name), a 28-year-old Hongkonger, completed his medical training in Ireland before returning to his home city in 2021. After a year of additional training, he began his career as a houseman* *at Princess Margaret Hospital in early 2022, just as Hong Kong was hit by the deadly fifth wave of the pandemic.*

'In Ireland, when I was on call, it was a 12-hour shift. In Hong Kong, I was doing 30-hour shifts. I was on the isolation wards. I'd start work on a Monday at 9 am, and the shift would end about 2 pm the next day. There was supposed to be time to sleep during the shift, but during the fifth wave there wasn't the chance. Princess Margaret is the designated infectious diseases centre, and many of the wards were turned into COVID wards. Every time we went on the ward, we had to gown up and then gown down. Physically, it was very tiring.

'As an intern, I did a lot of the blood taking and managed the communication between the family members and patients. It was very stressful. Most of the patients were elderly and needed oxygen. Their blood results were poor, and they needed antivirals and antibiotics. There wasn't much else we could do for them. Many of the patients were dying because of COVID. We became quite numb to it.

'I honestly had a really bad time. I felt I couldn't deal with it, and my mental health deteriorated. I experienced panic attacks for the first time and developed anxiety and depression. It was so bad that I'd wake up crying in the middle of my sleep. If I took time off, someone would have to cover for me, and that would put pressure on my colleagues. I didn't want to do that. I thought that if I told my supervisor, I would be seen as weak. If you make a big deal of it, you can have time off. A colleague did, and I heard so many speak negatively about him. The seniors looked down on him; they said he was making excuses and lazy. I decided not to tell my supervisor. I only told my fiancée, family, and closest friends.

'I pushed through, and in my time off I went to see a psychiatrist and was in therapy. Whenever I broke down at work, I called my fiancée or my parents. I needed to have a way to express how

I was feeling at that moment. There were ups and downs. Anxiety and depression fluctuate a lot, but at your lowest point you feel there is no way out. I was too overwhelmed with the pressure; I needed someone to lean on.

'Unfortunately, Chinese culture doesn't deal with mental health very nicely. I don't think it's just in hospitals or the medical field. A lot of industries in Hong Kong, especially those with Asian culture, are like that. We are essential workers, so if you take time off someone else has to fulfil your duty, which puts pressure on your colleagues. I understand that, but they should be more encouraging to talk about mental health. If we had been told at our orientation, "You will undergo a lot of stress. If you aren't feeling good, feel free to talk about it", then I'd have thought, "okay, you recognise this". But at my orientation all they said was, "It's going to be tough; good luck." There was no mention of mental health.

'I only found out much later that there was a mental health counsellor available for doctors as part of occupational health, but by then I was already dealing with it. Even if I'd wanted to, I didn't know how to contact that counsellor. There is a stigma that prevents people from going. Once you make a big deal of it, then your colleagues and seniors know. I really want to see change. It was the worst time in my life. Even months after the fifth wave, I'd get palpitations when I drove past the hospital.

'I am now a licensed doctor. COVID is over, so I don't get that kind of stress anymore, but I'm still taking medication. I used to say that I'd stay in the public system, but after what I experienced, I'm not sure. There is a real hierarchy in hospitals. The seniors have all the authority. You can't change things as a junior; you have to play the game. We were hit so badly by the fifth wave because the hospitals weren't open to change. They were so set in their way of doing things; they didn't want to talk about efficiency. I won't be one of those seniors. With the experience I have from the UK and Ireland, I will be more open about well-being and mental health. Hopefully, one day I will be senior enough to implement some sort of positive change.'

***Ka Po** (not her real name), a nurse at Princess Margaret Hospital in Kwai Chung in the New Territories, worked on the SARS wards in 2003, where she witnessed her colleagues succumb to the disease. When COVID-19 began, she knew she was potentially putting her life on the line. Her pandemic stresses came not from the virus but from despair at having to treat patients in tents on the street outside the hospital because the isolation wards were full.*

'I was a nurse during SARS. In the beginning, we didn't know what was happening. We thought it was something like a chest infection, but it turned out not to be. There were so many unknowns and uncertainties. We only had paper masks and certainly not full body cover. When I think back to that time, the thing that comes to me is the seriousness of the situation—the realisation that I could die from my work. A couple of my colleagues, a nurse and a doctor, passed away from SARS. When COVID came, it was all hands on deck because we knew people could die from it. We wondered whether this was going to be SARS 2, so we requested more protective equipment.

'In February 2020, just after Chinese New Year, there was a strike of medical workers. They were striking for the border with China to be closed to stop the virus coming into Hong Kong and for more PPE. I supported the strike, but I didn't join it because I'd already booked my vacation and was outside Hong Kong. When I got back to Hong Kong after my holiday, it was all hands on deck.

'Princess Margaret Hospital was the designated infection control centre, and a building was set aside for isolation wards. There were five floors for isolation wards, and the usual practice was to keep one floor empty for a real emergency as well as maintenance. My role is to assist the nurses who have recently graduated. I support them in their first year of their work. If they don't know the procedure, I tell them, and I offer psychological support.

'For the first half of 2020, we didn't have enough PPE and had to be really careful. We just had surgical masks and latex gloves for protection. It wasn't a good situation, but I was very cautious, and we managed. The instruction was to send COVID patients to isolation. If they weren't COVID positive, they went to the general ward. I was on the general ward, and some people were panicking because we were getting patients who tested positive one or two days after they were admitted, sometimes after just a few hours. From July onwards we had more PPE. The most worrying part for us was that the policy of the management changed daily, which kept us very busy transferring patients to different wards. In the am shift they might say, "Keep COVID patients in A&E." And on the pm shift they said, "Send them to isolation."

'On an isolation ward, we have a machine that creates negative pressure in the room, so that when the door is opened, contaminated air doesn't flow out. In 2021, the number of COVID cases increased in Hong Kong, so they changed the general ward into an isolation ward. We had three levels of ward: The most serious cases went to Block S, the infection control centre, which was level one. When that was full, a machine was used to turn the general ward into a negative-pressure ward, level two. And the third level, the surveillance ward, was a disaster because all the fever cases went there, but it didn't have negative pressure. I worked in levels one and two.

'Psychologically, the nurse students were okay, but the workload was really heavy. It was really tough. For my students, newly graduated nurses, it was mostly their parents who were worried about them working on the ward. Some of them quit because their families were worried. Overall, 2021 was still relatively stable. The challenges were mostly to do with the restrictions, the dining ban, and the lack of a social life. It got a lot more serious in 2022.

'We had to keep a 1.5-metre distance between COVID patients. During the fifth wave, the isolation wards filled up, so there were a lot of people outside the hospital because there wasn't room inside. Tents were put up outside the hospital, in the lane where the ambulances usually park, and it was turned into an outdoor ward. The ambulances had to park in the driving lane. It was chaotic. We had 30 to 40 patients lying on stretchers. In March [2022], my boss asked me to work in the tents outside. I felt as though I was working in a war zone.

'The situation for the patients was so poor. How can you put a patient in the street? We didn't have enough equipment. Some patients needed oxygen, but we didn't have enough. We had to use oxygen cylinders. When the cylinder gauge went into the red, showing that it was almost empty, we changed it. My colleagues told me that someone in senior management walked past the tent and saw them using bottled oxygen. That person said, "This is very expensive; don't change it until it's completely empty." We wondered what was going on. Hong Kong is an international city; how could we be in this situation?

'Most of the patients in the tents outside the hospital were elderly. We had just one or two nurses looking after 40 patients. We couldn't meet their daily care needs. Some patients were bedridden, and we had to change their diapers. This was all done outdoors. How could we keep their dignity?

'I wouldn't say that I was very stressed, but I found it tough. During work I was stressed. I'm used to shift work, but this was especially tiring. I'd get home at the end of a shift exhausted. My partner accepts that I work on the acute ward, that this is how my life is. I was so tired after a long shift that I'd fall asleep within five minutes; then I'd get up and go back to work.

'People who are struggling with their mental health can go to the Critical Incident Support Team where they have clinical psychologists and some volunteer staff. I was a volunteer staff member after SARS. If you feel depressed or need help, you can talk to them and have some counselling. But frankly, there's not much time for anyone to take it up.

'Hong Kong doesn't have enough hospitals and we don't have enough human resources or personnel. After SARS, we understood that another pandemic may come. Going through COVID with my colleagues, working together in the war zone, we've become very close. Like a firefighter who is always prepared for a fire, we nurses are always prepared. Psychologically, I'm prepared for another pandemic, but I don't know what we will face.'

***Bobo** (not her real name) has been working as a nurse in a public hospital in Hong Kong for nine years. Just before the pandemic hit, she was promoted to the position of 'IC' or the nurse in charge of a ward. In this role, she is responsible for overseeing all patients, as well as managing admissions and discharges.*

'When I went from being just a registered nurse to a more senior level, I took on a lot more responsibility and my stress increased. I was in charge of ward admission decisions, overseeing patients, and handing over to the next shift. We have six medical wards in our hospital. They transformed them progressively into COVID wards. I experienced many changes from a COVID ward back to a medical ward and then back to a COVID ward again. The first few times it was quite overwhelming. How do we arrange the equipment? How do we make the arrangements? My IC role together with COVID meant my stress was really intense. I'd say it was a 9 out of 10.

'I was on the dirty team with the COVID cases. I was with patients when the virus progressed suddenly, and they needed to be intubated and sent to the ICU. At the beginning of the pandemic, we didn't have enough PPE—masks, face shields, and that kind of thing. I felt like I was risking my life when I went to work. The hospital couldn't get supplies from the usual source and was getting PPE from mainland China, but there were lots of faults with it and it broke easily. In this profession, you know there will be risk, you expect it, but we felt helpless because we were not properly supported. We washed our hands as much as possible and tried to keep the equipment clean to protect ourselves and our patients. I wasn't afraid of the virus, but I was disappointed that we were so underprepared.

'Being on the COVID team I felt dirty. I didn't want to infect my family, so I moved out. Because I was working on the COVID ward, I could apply for an allowance of HK$500 a day for accommodation. I didn't have a social life during COVID. Even if I wanted to meet friends from outside, they might not want to have dinner with me because of the risk. Even at work we ate separately from others to reduce the risk. Many facilities were closed, and there wasn't much to do after work other than Netflix and sleep. Because of the intense pressure at work, I'd get back to my room very tired, but I didn't sleep well. I had no problem falling asleep because I was so exhausted, but

I'd wake up suddenly in the night worrying about something that had happened on my shift and wondering if I'd made a bad decision.

'The guidelines were very strict in the beginning, but then they kept changing and it was very difficult to follow them. There were many cases where I couldn't make a concrete decision based on the guidelines. Different wards were interpreting the guidelines differently. One moment things were very strict, and the next the guidelines collapsed and we didn't need to do all these tests. The guidelines weren't clear and didn't react to the situation. If I made a bad decision, I'd get blamed by my boss. That was the biggest pressure point for me and it made me quite angry.

'A number of times we had to quickly change a general ward into a COVID ward, but these wards couldn't support COVID patients; they didn't have negative pressure. Sometimes important treatments for our patients were missed. We had a renal case who was supposed to be in a renal ward, but they changed it into a COVID ward. I'm not saying the nurses weren't doing a good job, but they weren't used to looking after renal cases and weren't trained in kidney replacement therapy. It was super messy. The changes left us feeling helpless.

'In February and March 2022, our ward was super busy, and we couldn't accommodate all the cases. The pressure was super unbearable; the hospital just collapsed. It was so overwhelming. I'd never faced anything like that. I was quite new in my position as IC and I didn't want to piss off my boss or my colleagues. I wasn't worried about getting COVID; I was stressed about the changing hospital policy that we needed to follow. There were long queues of patients waiting for admission in the A&E. How could we transfer all these charges? How could we be quicker to admit the cases? When will the test results be available? The guidelines were not clear on things. If I made a wrong decision, my boss would ask me about it later.

'A shift is usually eight hours, but during COVID most of us worked overtime. My shift finished at 10 pm, but I often worked past midnight, and sometimes to 2 am. The nurses often missed dinner and kept on working. We didn't want to leave too much work unfinished for the night shift; there were only three people working the night shift. I really love my colleagues. If not for them, I don't think I could have stood that time. When we got a call from management asking for sudden changes, as IC I needed to tell them. Although they didn't want to do it, we worked together because we have such a good spirit and are good friends.

'The guidelines were issued by the Hospital Authority. Every hospital has an infection control team that monitors disease outbreaks like flu and COVID. This team advises on things such as which cases need to be put in an isolation room. The team goes off duty at 5 pm, but we work 24 hours a day. There was a lot of variety in the type of cases: quarantine cases, travelling cases, newly diagnosed cases, just-recovered cases, and readmission cases. If someone got COVID six months before and then they got it again, were they an old COVID patient or a new one? There was no clear definition on cases. As frontline staff, we were not certain about infection control policy; it kept changing. If we waited for the team to come on duty, it could be at the risk of our patients. You could play it safe and put the case in the isolation room, but that space is limited. What if you got a case that really needed isolation and there wasn't enough space?

'During the fifth wave, the infection control team did work 24 hours, but they were not very supportive of the night shift. COVID went on for three years. Where were they? They were supposed to react quickly, but I didn't see them doing an active job. My stress wasn't about COVID; it came from the guidelines which kept changing. More consistent and clear guidelines would have been better.

The government sent a representative to give us some biscuits, take a photo, and say they supported us. But I didn't feel supported.

'In the summer of 2022, I was working on the COVID ward when I tested positive for the virus. And then I discovered I was one-month pregnant. Pregnant nurses working on the COVID ward can choose to be moved to another ward. I decided to stay. I was familiar with running the ward, and had a good relationship with the team. I worked on the COVID ward through my pregnancy. My baby is now three months old, and I'm back at work. If not for my colleagues, I'd consider changing to a less stressful work environment, like an outpatient clinic. But because of them and the good atmosphere, I don't plan to quit. Work is stressful, but we share the workload and are friends; those relationships are invaluable.'

Tom *(not his real name) is a registered nurse. He completed his graduation in the midst of the pandemic and started his first job as a pre-registered nurse at Yan Chai Hospital, Tsuen Wan, in July 2021.*

'I studied nursing for five years. At university, they shared a bit about SARS. They told us to take precautions when handing airborne diseases, but they didn't talk about how to handle a pandemic. I was working on the general medical ward. The ward was full, and they added extra beds. To begin with I was looking after 8 to 12 patients and had time to chat to them and find out more about their condition. In February 2022, during the fifth wave, the workload was really high. I was looking after 15 to 17 patients. With that many patients, you can't remember all their names, and you may mix up patient A and patient B. The patient becomes an object; you don't have the time to spare to be with them and better understand their needs.

'The interaction with a patient is important in nursing, but there wasn't the time. If the patient had a complaint, I'd tell them that I would come back later, but I didn't have the time to go back. I barely had time to complete all the routine work on a shift. If I delayed my work, it would have to be passed over to other colleagues. During the pandemic, visitors weren't allowed. Some patients had been there two months. They hadn't seen their family, and they just lay in bed staring at the ceiling. I didn't have the time to take care of their emotional needs. Some patients may feel they'd been abandoned by their relatives. When the patient is very ill, or when they have passed away, we will call the family. The family would be crying a lot and blaming themselves for not being able to accompany the patient in the last stage of their life. I very nearly cried but managed to stop myself because I was working. My mood was very heavy; I felt very sad.

'The workload was so heavy, and you have to multitask. Under such stressful situations, sometimes I couldn't remember things so well and my colleagues would spot my mistake. Some colleagues are nice and speak to you privately if you miss something. But if my mistake got out and was known by the whole ward, then I felt very ashamed. When I left work, I'd feel very stressed and worry that I'd missed something. It would take a long time to fall asleep because I would be thinking about the scheduled treatment of my patient. The pressure and shame from the seniors was the most stressful part. Patients change, but my colleagues don't change so frequently.

'The hospital emailed us about a workshop on psychological support for frontline staff. I didn't go because I didn't want to be stigmatised. I was afraid that if I joined the course, I might be recognised and someone would think I was stressed and needed help. I don't know anyone who joined; none of my colleagues did. When I am stressed, I share it with my friends and family first.

'There is a lot of gossiping on the wards about the ability and character of colleagues, especially by the seniors. The senior staff have been working together for a long time, so they may have a close relationship. When I was new on the ward, I treated their opinion as a performance review.

'Some seniors are very strict and have high expectations of new staff. They assume that because they can do something you should be able to. If they offered to help staff, or talked about a problem privately rather than publicly, that would help new staff to grow. When you hear someone talking about you it makes you feel stressed. They might say, "Oh Tom left some work again; I have to pick things up." But you don't know what the problem is.

'During COVID I had to take care of many cases. When you see your colleagues can handle the job, you don't want to be the one to say, "I feel it is too stressful". I don't want to be gossiped about. If the seniors showed some understanding of the pressure that we were under during the pandemic, it would have made it less stressful. Every day I went onto the ward, I took a deep breath. It was like I was getting ready to go to hell.

'During COVID, I thought about switching to work in another environment, maybe an old age home. I think my resilience is much stronger than before, and I'm glad I'm still working at a public hospital. I have two friends who graduated in the same year as me. They went to work at Tuen Mun Hospital, and both quit after six months. They are now working in the private sector. If the whole culture in public hospitals could change, then more fresh graduates would stay in the public sector.'

***Jasmine Cheung**, a 30-year-old Chinese medicine practitioner, runs her own clinic in Prince Edward. She has observed an increase in the number of patients seeking help for mental health issues although many of them prefer not to be labelled as such.*

'In my industry, when people know you are a Chinese medicine practitioner, they and their friends and family want to find you; it's a kind of trust. At the start of the pandemic, I was working in a large clinic in a public hospital. The location wasn't favourable for everyone, so in my off time I secretly worked at my own small clinic. At the hospital, I needed to deal with 40 to 50 patients a day. There were always many patients waiting outside. I didn't have much time with each patient, which made work very stressful for me.

'The hospital implemented many restrictions on patients, including a very strict body temperature control. They set up a high-risk team and assigned one doctor to deal with all the people with a high temperature. A high temperature can mean any number of illnesses. Chinese medicine is different from Western medicine because we have a flow with our patients; different doctors use different methods. The policy meant that our long-term patients couldn't find us. It was a ridiculous system because the doctor assigned to high temperature cases changed every day, so that in itself was risk. We tried to talk to the management team about the ridiculous policy, but they didn't listen. They didn't have a medical background; they were just management people. Many of my colleagues and I didn't feel good about working there so we left.

'During the first and second waves of COVID in the first half of 2020, I went to stay at my grandpa's place in the countryside in Taiwan. I did video sessions with my patients. In the past, we didn't offer online treatment partly because it wasn't covered by insurance. But the insurance policy was changed during COVID; it was a remarkable change. Particularly later in the pandemic, when the mainstream service couldn't manage the number of cases, more people turned to Chinese medicine. Our industry developed a rapid delivery service to get herbal medicine to patients within a day. In rural Taitung, people weren't wearing masks, and I felt quite distant from the situation in Hong Kong. I felt quite sad and helpless listening to my patients in Hong Kong.

'When I returned to Hong Kong, I continued doing video sessions and switched to in-person when the restrictions allowed. In my own clinic, I could work at my own pace. Although a lot of my patients were unstable, I felt like I had the time and was capable of dealing with them because I could work at my own rhythm. I didn't have to give them signals to end the session, and we could talk and let the emotion flow.

'I have noticed that more of my patients are showing signs of mental health issues, but many of them are not admitting that. Often when they come to a Chinese medicine doctor, they don't want a concrete diagnosis on their mental health issues. They don't want to be labelled. We talk about other symptoms like a headache, stomachache, or low mood. In our approach, we may have a diagnosis that is 90 percent the same as depression, but because they have other symptoms, we take it as a whole. In Chinese medicine, we treat the person as a whole. I think they are more comfortable with that. Our medicine can help them reduce their low mood.

'Many people had emotional breakdowns in the video consultations. They talked about how they couldn't go out and couldn't meet their family and friends. The elderly homes weren't allowing visitors, and many people hadn't seen their parents for a long time. One of my patients, a guy who worked in IT, was so desperate to see his mother that he was even talking about getting a job in his mother's care home so he could see her. Eventually, the staff at the care home set up a call for him. His mother's Alzheimer's had worsened, and she didn't recognise him. He was devastated and cried and cried. It was upsetting for us both. I couldn't do anything about his situation, but I felt that being with him was of some help. At least he knew someone was listening.

'Chinese medicine develops from the theory that there are internal and external reasons for disease. Internal are related to extreme emotions—too sad or too nervous—and external might be bacteria or a virus. The internal reasons are really important to understand why a person is getting ill. I spend a lot of time talking to my patients about their situation. The conversation will often go deep, which perhaps make me sound like a counsellor.

'When I began seeing patients in person, I didn't put a plexiglass screen between us. I touched their hand to check their pulse and looked into their eyes. For many people during the pandemic, especially the elderly, seeing the doctor was a good excuse to go out. For some of them it had been a long time since someone had touched them or spoken to them without a plexiglass screen between them. I felt like I was providing a meaningful service.

'One of my patients is a six-year-old boy. After three years of online lessons and on and off schooling, he finally went back to school and played with his friends. He's a normal kid and plays with my staff when he comes to the clinic. Because he's been at home for three years, his immune system is weak, and he gets sick easily. His symptoms don't last long, and he is strong enough to overcome it, but his parents are extremely nervous and bring him to the clinic every week. I've tried to explain to them that this is normal, and he needs to build up his immune system, but they keep taking him out of school for a week at a time. This is the parents' anxiety affecting the child.

'I've known many of my patients a long time and know them quite well. I can see that the pandemic has changed them a lot. They don't know what they should do, what they are allowed to do, and are constantly confused. The policy was really strict, and it became a habit to stick to it, even though the policy itself was often unclear and difficult to follow. It's as though the part of their mind related to COVID-19 is messed up and doesn't connect with their logical, rational brain. Even though the restrictions have been lifted, they are still giving off a nervous vibe.'

* * *

In Hong Kong, we knew from the experience of SARS in 2003 that working in tense conditions and under extreme stress puts front-line medical workers at risk of anxiety, insomnia, and fatigue in the short term. In the long term, they are at risk of underlying illness, PTSD, and burnout. Studies after the SARS epidemic showed that 90 percent of the city's healthcare professionals with high-exposure risk in clinical settings reported mental health problems. After SARS, nurses reported increased levels of anxiety, depression, and PTSD (Thompson et al., 2004).

Reflecting on the lessons learned from SARS, Robert Maunder, professor of psychiatry at the University of Toronto, wrote in 2009: 'Now that we know more about the psychological impact of a dramatic outbreak of infectious disease, we are in a much better position to prepare effectively for future events. Now is the time to build the resilience of healthcare workers and healthcare organisations in order to reduce the impact of pandemic influenza or other unforeseen outbreaks' (Maunder, 2009).

Sound advice, but it didn't happen in Hong Kong. Despite the earlier experience of SARS, healthcare workers during the COVID-19 pandemic were left without adequate resources and psychological support.

The city's healthcare system was grappling with a shortage of hospital beds, scant resources, and a lack of staff long before COVID-19 (Cheung & Yip, 2015). The health authorities had been warning for years about a staffing shortage, predicting a shortfall of 1,610 doctors by the end of the decade, rising to 1,949 by 2040 (Lam, 2021).

Healthcare workers were already under pressure, and the pandemic restrictions meant they were expected to respect social distancing as much as possible. The disruption of routines and interaction led to social isolation, which reduced the degree of social support that is one of the main sources of stress reduction. This led to poor mental health and an increase in burnout.

Burnout is a type of exhaustion that appears after people have been constantly experiencing anxiety and stress. It can cause people to lose interest in their work and fail to see its value. Health workers in Hong Kong were particularly susceptible to burnout due to the drawn-out nature of the pandemic, which lasted for three years and affected the city in successive waves.

A study conducted in 2022 found that nurses in Hong Kong experienced significant psychological distress during the city's deadly fifth wave of the pandemic. The study revealed that nurses felt exhausted, stressed, depressed, worried, frustrated, and fearful. Their fear was largely attributed to their close contact with infected patients and the increased stress of caring for confirmed cases. The study also identified several other factors contributing to their distress, including insufficient resources such as isolation facilities and PPE, low job satisfaction, and a lack of organisational support (Cheung et al., 2023).

Frontline medical workers were particularly concerned about the possibility of bringing the virus home and infecting their loved ones. Their fears were well founded, as a study by Shah et al. (2020) found that the risk of hospitalisation during the pandemic was three times higher for healthcare professionals and twice as high for their household members compared to the general population.

Frontline medics are often praised as heroes and commended for 'soldiering on' in the face of adversity. While this recognition is well intentioned, the use of heroic narratives and militaristic metaphors can make it difficult for them to admit when they are struggling. Healthcare workers may feel that expressing emotions is unprofessional or a sign of weakness. Despite the general agreement that mental health support is desirable, research suggests that there is a reluctance to seek help (Billings et al., 2021). Fearing the stigma associated with experiencing stress and mental health issues, many healthcare workers may choose to suffer in silence. Concerns about confidentiality and the potential impact on their careers can also deter them from seeking support, leading to an over-reliance on self-treatment, inadequate peer support, and an increased risk of suicide.

Nurses in Hong Kong have been facing high levels of stress in the workplace. A survey conducted between April and June 2020 found that nearly 80 percent of the 854 nurses interviewed reported moderate to high levels of perceived stress. Additionally, 50.9 percent of the nurses were found to have symptoms of PTSD (Xie et al., 2021). A subsequent study conducted two years later revealed that nurses continued to experience significant psychological distress and reported a lack of support in coping with the challenges of working in a high-pressure and high-risk environment (Cheung et al., 2023).

Providing psychological support for frontline healthcare workers is essential. However, the question remains: How can it be provided in a way that is sensitive and effective? A review of 46 qualitative studies exploring healthcare workers' experiences of pandemics and epidemics, including COVID-19, found some common ground. Healthcare workers responded well to training when it was practical and specific. They valued clear, consistent, and compassionate communication from their organisations. When their safety was prioritised and they were supported with manageable workloads and time out from work, they felt valued by their employers. They also wanted to be consulted and included in decision-making. The value of peer support and emotional guidance from colleagues cannot be understated. This points to possible opportunities to further develop peer support systems and increase mental health awareness in the workplace (Billings et al., 2021).

The strategies outlined below can help healthcare workers support their mental health, but it is clear that organisations and the government must provide support. It is not sustainable to place the burden on healthcare workers to recognise and monitor their own stress and burnout. During a crisis, medical professionals are focused on saving lives, and it is only after the immediate threat has passed that the true cost on mental health emerges. Now, in the aftermath of the COVID-19 pandemic, we must not only recognise its impact on mental health but also put systems in place to enable a solid recovery and ensure we are prepared for the next pandemic.

Strategies and Support

Self-care / Health care professionals are trained to prioritise patients' needs. However, they may not always prioritise their own self-care due to fear of judgment from others or feeling selfish. Practising self-care is crucial for coping with the demands of their profession and achieving a better balance between work and personal life. It can also help protect their health, well-being, and job satisfaction.

- **Spiritual practices and relaxation techniques** can help you find inner peace and calmness. You might consider trying yoga, meditation, or deep-breathing exercises. Take time to do simple actions that bring joy, comfort, and boost your self-esteem.
- **E-mental health services** are a great way to get professional help and support for your mental health. You can access them from the comfort of your own home.
- **Interpersonal skills** are important for building strong relationships with others. You can practise active listening, empathy, and effective communication. Communicate openly with your supervisor and ask for the support you need.
- **Prioritising close relationships** such as those with family can help you feel more connected and supported. You might consider creating a platform, either formal or informal, where you and your colleagues can discuss challenges and share knowledge.
- **Maintaining a healthy lifestyle** by maintaining a healthy diet, ensuring adequate sleep and regular exercise can help you feel more energised and refreshed.
- **Enjoying recreational activities and hobbies** can help you find joy and fulfilment in life.

Mindfulness is an evidence-based approached that can help you stay present in the moment and reduce stress. It has been proven to decrease burnout and improve mental well-being among healthcare providers (Goodman & Schorling, 2012). Interventions incorporating elements of mindfulness can increase resilience, alleviate fatigue and burnout, and nurture psychological well-being. You might connect to your senses to bring you fully into the moment. Begin by noticing what you see, and then focus in turn on what you can hear, smell, and feel. This simple practice will help to ground you fully in the present and calm your mind.

7

Child Separation

In early 2022, Hong Kong was gripped by fear as children who tested positive for COVID-19 were forcibly separated from their parents. This policy sent shockwaves throughout the city, causing local parents to become hesitant to take their children to hospital for fear of being separated. For many expatriate families, this was the final straw, and they decided to leave Hong Kong permanently.

*In February 2022, **Laura Hazlett**, a 32-year-old first-time mother, faced a difficult situation when her 11-month-old daughter, Ava, fell ill with a high fever. Acting on her doctor's advice, Laura, who is a communications professional, and her husband took Ava to Queen Mary Hospital for treatment.*

'Things had kicked off in Hong Kong and lots of people had COVID. It felt as if it was closing in on us. Then our helper got it, and on the Sunday, Ava started coughing. I had lots of friends in the UK who had been through COVID with kids and everything was fine, so I wasn't too worried. That night Ava got a lot worse; she had a fever of 40 degrees and was really unsettled. We moved a mattress into her room and slept with her. I'd had Ava at the Matilda, and I called the hospital to get advice. They said that if she has COVID and her condition worsens to take her to a public hospital.

'On the Monday, Ava was quite lethargic, lying on us, which was unusual because she's usually active. I called Central Health [Medical Practice] and did a video consult with the paediatrician. The doctor asked to see Ava's chest and stomach. She said she was worried about Ava's breathing and advised us to call an ambulance. She said if her oxygen levels were high, she wasn't too worried, but to check.

'We live in Sai Ying Pun, so Queen Mary is the obvious hospital to go to. We called an ambulance, and they said it would be a four- to five-hour wait, so we threw a bag together and got a taxi. We knew about the hysteria about COVID, that we'd probably be quarantined, and it would be a long process, but I assumed I'd be able to stay with her.

'We got to Queen Mary at midday. They saw us straight away and checked her temperature and oxygen levels. Her oxygen was fine. Then they took her to X-ray her chest and lungs. We were told she'd go to the paediatric ward and only one parent could go with her. I went with her and we were put in an isolation room—a big empty room with just one bed. The paediatrician was young and wasn't empathetic or kind. He gave her a steroid shot and a COVID test. I was there for hours and hours while Nick was standing in a corridor somewhere. I asked if my husband could come in the room, but was told no.

'At 10.30 pm Ava's COVID test came back positive. The doctor said, "You are a close contact, so you need to isolate for 14 days." I pleaded to go outside and speak to my husband, but the doctor said, "You must go home. I want to transfer Ava to the ICU. You need to leave."

'I was going from hysteria and crying, to angry, to being firm and fair and understanding, and then pleading. I was an absolute mess. It was a blur. As a parent it was very stressful choosing between getting my child the help she needed and being separated. I asked if we could discharge Ava—I just wanted to know if we could—and was told that now she was a confirmed case she needed to be there for seven days.

'We got in the lift with Ava to take her to the ICU. She was crying, distressed, disorientated, and not feeling well. I didn't want to leave her. The doctor said, "You need to leave. If you don't, I'm going to call security and they'll call the police." My husband left an iPad with the nurse so we could communicate with her.

'It was really hard, and I sobbed in the taxi home. At 4 am we called the hospital and they said she was sleeping, which gave us some comfort. She was obviously sick, but it was more the fact I wasn't with her. In the morning, I spoke to a lovely doctor who was empathetic, and that helped so much. She explained the rules were changing constantly and now the best-case scenario was we'd see her in seven days. She wasn't telling us anything different, but she empathised with us and said, "I'm so sorry you're going through this; this is awful. I want you to know Ava is doing well." The kindness and empathy changed the whole outlook the next day. I felt relief that someone knew what was going on and would advocate for me, Ava, and Nick. I didn't feel that first doctor was on our side. He wasn't clear about the next steps or how long she would be there.

'I wanted to go to the hospital, but as we were close contacts we had to self-isolate. I was feeling like the worst possible mum because I was away from my child. She was 10 minutes down the road, and I couldn't see her or be with her. By Wednesday, Nick and I were both testing positive on RAT tests and coughing. Ava was stable and we were given two options: to go with Ava to Penny's Bay, not knowing how long we'd be there, or to wait until she was released on Monday. I couldn't wait until Monday; we needed Ava back. To prove that we had COVID, we had to get a PCR test from an official testing centre, but when we got to the centre they wouldn't let us in because we had symptoms. We called Queen Mary and said, "This is ridiculous, they won't accept us because we've got symptoms." We were told, "Ok, don't worry about getting tested."

'We were escorted by security guards to a special lift and waited an hour to get into the paediatric ward. Ava was wheeled out in a cot. She was wearing a baby shield and crying. She didn't understand what was going on. We got on a bus to Penny's Bay. We were so happy to be together but had no idea how long we'd be at the quarantine centre. In the end, we spent three days there and were released when we showed three negative tests. We had a bit of Stockholm syndrome and felt we were lucky to get out after three days.

'We had so many friends here with children who fled Hong Kong because they were petrified that would happen to them. A friend had a daughter the same age as Ava who tested positive. She went to Queen Mary, but she wouldn't let her be admitted because she was so worried about being separated from her. People were saying, "We will keep our children at home and not take them to hospital for fear of the consequences." It was hard for us because we were in it, but it was hard for every parent in Hong Kong. If it had happened to a friend of ours, I'd have found it traumatic.

'I have changed off the back of that. Day to day I'm fine; I've moved past it, but with the girls I have really bad health anxiety about them being ill. It's really triggering to me if the girls are sick. I don't know if we'll ever forgive Hong Kong for what it did, but I recognise it was a mad time. I'm sure if it happened again it would be different. We were caught up in a mess.'

In March 2022, **Arlene***, a first-time mother, took her 21-month-old daughter to the hospital for a routine check-up. However, she was shocked when she was informed that her daughter would have to stay overnight and that she wouldn't be allowed to stay with her. After her daughter was released following a traumatic four-day stay, Arlene left a distraught message in the comments section of the* South China Morning Post, *alongside a story on child separation.*

'My daughter has just been discharged from the hospital this afternoon. At first, we only brought her for a check-up for a swollen hand from a possible insect bite. After waiting for a few hours at the A&E, the doctor told us that she needed to be admitted. Of course, as her mother, I strongly said no, and so did my husband because we were told we wouldn't be able to visit her, and I couldn't stay with her. She's only 21 months. What an abuse.

'The next day they called and told us that she tested positive for COVID-19. How did that happen? We did an antigen test at home, and both my husband and I are negative. While our daughter was in hospital, they gave us updates, telling us that she was eating well, drinking lots of liquid, and playing with the nurses.

'Finally, after four days, the hospital called and said she could be discharged. My husband picked her up. She has lost weight, her knees and legs are weak, her voice is weak, and I can tell that she has been crying a lot. Even her eyes seem very sleepy. Seeing her, I almost cried my eyes out. She has severe skin rashes. I guess they didn't check her diapers regularly.

'She came home with a different attitude. Whenever she cries, she slaps her tummy or hurts me. And my child used to be a very sweet baby. She's grumpy and often shouts out, "No!" That makes me think that they might have shouted at her in the hospital when she fought back against tests and medications that they administered.

'As a mother it really pains to see this happen to my child who is still a baby. They separated me from her. You people are giving our children severe trauma. It's very abusive for them. I don't know where to start or how to comfort her from what she has gone through. It's a nightmare for every parent. I hope someone out there will do something about this situation.'

* * *

Dr Lucy Lord, executive chair of the mental health charity MIND Hong Kong, estimated that between 1,000 and 2,000 children infected with COVID-19 were separated from their parents in the six weeks leading up to the end of March 2022 (Sun, 2022). Some of these children were infants, and more than 90 percent of them were from local Chinese families. The Hospital Authority did not maintain official statistics on child separation cases during the so-called 'fifth wave' of the pandemic. A request for data on this issue received the following response from the Hospital Authority: 'The HA does not compile the information. According to paragraph 1.14 of the Code on Access to Information, the Code does not oblige departments to create a record which does not exist.'

For many parents, the fear of being separated from their children or having their children face quarantine or hospitalisation alone was greater than their fear of the virus itself. The American, British, and Australian consulates all issued statements warning against travel to Hong Kong due to the risk of parents being separated from their children as a result of COVID-19 infections. During the fifth wave, which saw the highest number of infections, the hospital system was under immense pressure and severely understaffed. There were reports of children being left alone in hospital wards, some getting their limbs stuck in cots and suffering accidents.

The scientific evidence against separating children from their parents is overwhelming. Separation can have devastating short-term and long-term impacts on a child's mental and physical well-being. Children, especially younger ones, depend on their parents for emotional support and well-being. Parents play a crucial role in promoting their child's healthy development and protecting them from the psychological consequences of stress, by helping them regulate their emotions. Separation from a parent can be traumatic and have detrimental behavioural and biological consequences for children and adolescents, even years later (Schraedley et al., 2002).

In early 2022, there were heart-wrenching scenes of children who tested positive for COVID-19 being forcibly separated from their parents by hospital staff in full protective gear, both the mother and child screaming in protest. When a child is separated under such chaotic circumstances, the brain and the body are flooded with stress hormones such as cortisol and adrenaline. In the short term, these hormones help the body cope with the immediate stress, but when present in high doses over an extended time, they can cause toxic stress that disrupts brain development and increases the risk of cognitive impairment and stress-related diseases later in life. Research has shown that children who experience such traumatic events can suffer from symptoms of anxiety and PTSD (Hornor, 2015).

Toxic stress can have a lasting impact on a child's brain. According to a study by Shonkoff et al. (2012), children who experience toxic stress may become visibly distressed and eventually become quiet and withdrawn. This is not that they have adapted to the situation but rather that their cortisol levels have been depleted and their stress response has been impaired. The researchers found that this can lead to a weak foundation for future learning, behaviour, and health.

The emotional bond that a child forms with their primary caregiver is crucial for their development. In 1969, British psychoanalyst John Bowlby proposed the attachment theory, suggesting that the first 2.5 years of a child's life are critical for forming this bond. A secure attachment allows the child to trust their caregiver, express their emotions, and eventually trust others, providing a strong foundation for healthy relationships in the future. However, if this primary bond is not formed or is disrupted, it can result in an insecure attachment and lead to anxiety and other mental health issues.

A study conducted by Howard et al. (2011) found that children who were separated from their mothers for a week or more during their first two years of life experienced distress due to their lack of cognitive abilities to understand the continuity of maternal availability. For three-year-olds, this separation was associated with increased negativity towards their mother, while children aged three to five were found to exhibit more aggression towards that parent.

However, the negative impact of separation is not limited to the child. For parents, few events are as traumatic as being separated from their child. During the Hong Kong pandemic, these emotions were likely intensified by the climate of fear and uncertainty, even after being reunited with their child.

Hong Kong boasts an excellent medical system, with doctors and nurses who understand the potential dangers and harm caused by separating a child from their parents. However, during the most chaotic period of the pandemic, the immediate risk of virus transmission was deemed more important than the long-term health and well-being of children and their parents.

Strategies and Support / How to Support Your Child and Yourself during Separation

If possible, maintain daily contact with your child through virtual calls and messages. This may involve leaving an iPad or other device with your child or, if they are very young, with hospital staff. Although it can be challenging, it is important to remain calm and composed, avoiding any signs of distress. Encourage your child to share their experiences and feelings by asking open-ended, non-judgemental questions such as 'Can you tell me about what you're doing?' or 'How does that make you feel?' and actively listen to their responses. While it may be tempting to jump into problem-solving mode, it is more important at this stage to ensure that your child feels heard and understood. Listen attentively to what they say and validate their emotions by saying things like, 'it's okay to feel angry right now'.

Being separated from your child can be an incredibly distressing experience for a parent. It's important to be kind to yourself and look after your own well-being during this difficult time. Ensuring that you get enough sleep and eat a healthy diet can help you maintain resilience, so you will be better able to support your child. It's also important to have someone to confide in, whether it's a partner, close friend, or therapist. Sharing your concerns and fears with someone you trust can help prevent your emotions from escalating and provide you with much-needed support.

When you are reunited with your child, let them know that you love them and are there to support them. Reassure them that they are safe and that the separation was not their fault. Resuming your usual home routine, including meals, bedtime, and other activities, can help your child feel secure again. If they are ready to talk, encourage them to share their experiences and validate their feelings. If they are reluctant to talk, give them space and let them know that you are there for them whenever they are ready.

Although your child might say they are fine, keep a close eye out for signs that they may be struggling. Behaviours such as increased clinginess or anxiety, more frequent or explosive meltdowns, withdrawal, repeatedly re-enacting the event, and bedwetting can all indicate that your child is having difficulty processing what happened. If they don't show signs of improvement, seek help from your GP or paediatrician as soon as possible. The earlier you reach out for help, the better.

Even after being reunited with your child, you may find that your thoughts are racing and you are experiencing feelings of panic. Taking a few moments to do a simple breathing exercise can help calm your mind and body. Inhaling deeply activates the sympathetic nervous system, which controls the fight-or-flight response, while exhaling activates the parasympathetic nervous system, which helps the body relax and calm down.

1. Sit comfortably with a straight back and close your eyes. Breathe through your nose.
2. Inhale for a count of two, then pause at the top of your inhale for a count of one.
3. Exhale gently for a count of four, then pause at the bottom of your exhale for a count of one. Keep your breathing even and smooth.
4. Repeat this exercise for at least five minutes, then check in with yourself and see if you notice a difference in your mood.
5. If the two-four count feels too short, you can increase the length of your breaths to four in and six out or six in and eight out. The key is that the exhale is longer than the inhale.

8

Pilots

The global aviation industry was severely affected by the pandemic. Flight crews worldwide faced reduced salaries, furloughs, or layoffs, and those who retained their jobs had to work in significantly altered environments with added stressors. The situation was particularly challenging for pilots based in Hong Kong, which implemented some of the strictest coronavirus regulations globally. The prolonged duration of the pandemic, coupled with the rigorous testing and quarantine protocols, resulted in extremely demanding working conditions.

In early 2021, Hong Kong classified many destinations, including Britain and the United States, as 'high-risk' countries. As a result, pilots flying passengers inbound from those countries were required to undergo a two-week—and later a three-week—hotel quarantine. In order to staff those flights, Cathay Pacific began running 'closed loop' rosters on a voluntary basis in February 2021. This required pilots to work for 21 days on a continuous loop, being shuttled between the airport and a quarantine hotel. Afterward, they would spend two weeks in a quarantine hotel before being released for two weeks of leave. In this way, many pilots spent months in isolation without access to fresh air or a gym.

***John** (not his real name), a freight pilot in his 30s, works for an airline based in Hong Kong. Throughout the pandemic, he transported cargo, including vaccines, medicine, and supplies, into the city. John got married in his native Malaysia in late 2019. When the border closed in March 2020, he was based in Hong Kong and accepted the strict measures, assuming they would be temporary. However, two years into the pandemic there was no end in sight for the restrictions. He badly missed his wife and family, and his mental health began to suffer as a result.*

'The closed loop arrangement meant that for six weeks at a time we were shuttled between the airport and hotels. It was really strict in Hong Kong—we were taken on a bus from the aircraft to the hotel and from the hotel straight to the aircraft. All along we were monitored. They put cable ties on the bus to and from the hotel to make sure we couldn't get out. They treated us like animals. Everyone was drained and borderline depressed.

'After we landed and did a PCR test, we had to get a document that said we were under medical surveillance. At one point they even put GPS trackers on us. My entire life was focused on meeting the restrictions. It messes with you mentally and you keep second-guessing self, wondering, "Have I done something wrong?" I can honestly tell you that none of us were 100 percent focused when flying these planes. We were focused on when we would see our families and when this would end.

'When there was no sign of it letting up, it got really ugly. A lot of scrutiny was placed on the flight crew, and we were blamed for the fifth wave outbreak, which wasn't true. The media went to town with it. After the article about the two Cathay crew going out and being responsible for the outbreak, we couldn't go out without getting unwanted attention. I called a taxi to go to work and when the driver saw me, he turned around. I got on a bus and sat at the back. People took one look at me and moved to the front of the bus. For the first time in my career, I was ashamed to wear my uniform.

'We were totally cut off from the outside world. It got dangerous when we accepted that this is what it was going to be. All those restrictions were for nothing. I don't feel it was a matter of public health or saving lives; it was just a matter of being seen to do things. None of the policymakers think of mental health.

'One of my colleagues landed and tested positive at the airport. After 12 hours waiting in the airport for the documentation to come through and the right transport, he was shipped off to Penny's Bay like a diseased animal. When he came out after 21 days, he was angry all the time. His mindset was muddled. From what I saw, no one was focused on the flying. Granted it was a routine procedural job, but there will always be that one day when something goes wrong, and that's when the spare brain capacity comes in. It was reduced for all of us.

'A lot of my colleagues have left Hong Kong. I almost left but decided to stay. For me honestly, I still feel the effects of it. I'm not the same person I used to be. I don't go out much. I don't meet people much. I stay at home in my safe place and avoid crowded places. Going to work with this thing over your head, it made the flying environment unsafe. All people were talking about was when would we see our families and whether we'd be retrenched. All the spare brain capacity we should have had to focus on flight safety was being used up worrying what about would happen to us.

'The airline says they will offer support, but it's a double-edged sword. If you are a pilot and getting mental help, when the word gets out you could be grounded. Everyone in this industry is scared of that, which is why no one spoke out. It is a huge safety issue which no one talks about. If you talk to your manager, he will say why not take six months of unpaid leave. I couldn't afford to do that.

'In the beginning it was fine; we accepted that we needed to do our part to help the government. But it got worse and worse. From the company perspective, they could have said, "If you want to get help, we will get you help with no repercussions." From a government perspective, they didn't need to be so harsh with us. They could have shown us more trust. In this industry we are responsible. Our job depends on adhering to policy and following procedures. Being made to wear a wrist tag at home and having to report all our activities created an additional level of stress.'

***David** (not his real name) is a pilot in his 40s with Cathay Pacific's passenger fleet. When he landed at Chek Lap Kok Airport in March 2020, he had no idea that he wouldn't fly again until December 2021. Unable to work, he found himself caught in limbo. The stress of job insecurity, loneliness, and missing his family in the UK made this the darkest period in his life.*

'Flying got less and less as Cathay began winding down, and then the brakes went on completely and I didn't fly for 21 months. Even now [April 2023] there are guys who still haven't been reactivated after three years. The company asked us to take a 15 percent temporary pay cut for six months. Then they changed everyone's contract to expire on December 31, 2021, and said if we didn't sign a new contract by January 1 we'd be out of a job. They cancelled my contract. I got a 40 percent pay cut and they reduced my pension and health benefits. The roster came out on the 15th of every month, so you knew the following month whether you were flying. Even though I wasn't working, I couldn't leave Hong Kong, because returning from the UK would have meant a 21-day washout in another country and then a 21-day quarantine when I got to Hong Kong. I kept thinking, "Cathay can't keep paying me for much longer".

'People would say you got paid 80 percent of your salary all that time and you didn't lift a finger; it sounds great. But it's not. I was worried about my job all the time, wondering where else I could get an aviation job. I was sitting on my own at home on Christmas Day 2020, not knowing if my job was safe and thinking, "What am I doing?" I was miserable and lonely. If I'd been told I'd be in the same situation a year later, I'd have left. I put on my trainers and walked out the door. I walked 20 km—to the Big Buddha and up Sunset Peak. The countryside and my mountain bike saved me. If it wasn't for walking and hiking, I wouldn't be here.

'I'd meet up with my friends and we were all in the same predicament. It's the most miserable drink because everyone is venting, but if you don't vent and you bottle it up you will implode. The wife of one of my best friends returned to Hong Kong with their 8-year-old daughter. The girl tested positive at the airport, and they snatched her from her mum. They were both screaming, and they tore them apart. They put his wife in Penny's Bay and took the little girl to hospital. They had no contact with the girl for 14 days. They only found out after she was released that people in hazmat suits had done anal and vaginal swabs on their little girl. The parents never gave their consent; they were never asked. His wife and daughter left Hong Kong; they'll never come back. That made me so angry, I saw red. How could they do that to a child? I'm not an angry or a violent person, but I've never been angrier in my life. I saw a lot of arguments in the bars where guys would snap; everyone was on edge. One of my friends committed suicide—he was doing the closed loops. Apart from the one day out to fly, he was locked up. Once you are in the closed loop you can't get out of it.

'I went for two years and four months of not seeing my family in the UK. The only way I could see them was to go sick. I went to an aviation doctor and told him I wasn't fit to fly mentally. When you get signed off as aero medically unfit, they don't say why. They don't say you are just sad and miserable and want to see your family; they treat you as if you have mental issues. The people making the rules all have their families here. Ninety-five percent of us did it because it was the only way to see our families, and 99 percent of us came back from seeing family feeling refreshed. Once you're signed off, it is a nightmare to get your license again. When I came back, I had to see a doctor, then a psychologist, then an aviation doctor and then the HK CAD [Civil Aviation Department].

'When I began flying after 21 months, everything had changed. There was a lot more paperwork; it was like starting new. Every time I went to work, I didn't know if I'd get locked up at Penny's Bay when I came back. My first flight was an 11-hour flight from Frankfurt. I landed in Hong Kong and then sat on a plastic chair for nine hours waiting to get my PCR test result. They began doing a 21-day look-back. It meant that if someone tested positive, they also locked up anyone who had been in contact with them over the past 21 days. A pilot friend flew to Sydney. One of the cabin crew tested positive, so they all got sent to Penny's Bay. They also sent my friend's wife and kids to Penny's Bay. It didn't make any sense—he hadn't seen them since he came into contact with the positive cabin crew. There was a lack of common sense. That's why everyone was so angry.'

***Barry** (not his real name), an Australian freight pilot in his late 40s, was working for Cathay Pacific during the pandemic. In the two and a half years before he left the airline in August 2022, he estimates he underwent more than 1,000 PCR tests and stopped counting his cumulative days in quarantine when he reached 200. Due to lengthy quarantine regulations in both Hong Kong and Australia, he didn't see his children in Australia for two years.*

'I was on the 747, which was only freight. As the world went into lockdown, it shifted quickly from normal operations, to suggesting that we don't go out, to telling us we can't go out. Fairly soon we were told we had to stay in our hotel rooms. We'd fly to a place and be transported to the hotel and then from the hotel back to the plane. You couldn't go out to exercise or get food.

'Flying cargo, every month was like pre-Christmas; we were super busy. The flight patterns became quite inefficient. If there wasn't another freight flight going the next day, you had to stay in the hotel room until there was one. We often waited a week, and the longest I waited was nine days.

'As restaurants shut down, we lived on a diet of delivered pizzas. It was months before Deliveroo, or the equivalent, ramped up. It's wasn't healthy. It was insidious and it got worse over time. It affected my physical health because I was so sedentary. I put on 10 kg in first year. After my annual medical, I got a letter from the Civil Aviation Department saying that my BMI was too high. I was given a year to lose the weight. There was no acknowledgment that we weren't able to exercise. One of my colleagues put on 25 kg and was told to lose it.

'I had a couple of toothaches. The dentist required that I be in the country for two weeks before I could get an appointment, but I couldn't get the time off work to meet that requirement. When I eventually went to get my teeth fixed after three years, the dentist said they weren't fixable, and I ended up losing three teeth.

'It is very weird being locked away from people for extended periods. You don't see your family, don't have your normal social interactions. Unlike my friends in other industries, the most normal part of my life was when I was at work. Once we got on the plane, the doors were closed, and it was just the crew. We took our masks off because we needed to be able to put on oxygen masks in case of depressurization. When I got to the other end and put on the parking break, I had a sinking feeling because I knew I was going to get locked up again.

'I had a serious family emergency with one of my kids in Australia. My medical examiner in Hong Kong said I wasn't fit to fly while I was dealing with that and signed me off for a couple of months. The time off was tied to my mental state and the stress factor; it was the doctor's decision. The two months was to give me time to get to Australia, deal with it, and travel back with the long quarantines. The problem with mental issues and fatigue is it's hard to judge. The people who need to make those decisions are the pilots themselves, and you make the worst decisions when you are fatigued and under stress.

'At that time in the freight world, we were short of pilots. I know of people who tried to be pre-emptive and said, "I need six months off to sort some things out." And they couldn't get it. The word filtered out that you needed to get your medical examiner to say you are unfit, but most of us considered there was a risk that once that happened you may lose your medical certification and then couldn't work. If you are refused a medical certificate in one country, you can try asking for one in another county, but there's a risk you might be out of the industry. A lot of people took the view that it was better to leave and start somewhere else than take the risk. Cathay was good in dealing with us as employees, but they were stuck between the demands of the Hong Kong government and what was possible and safe to do.

'There were probably about 3,000 freight pilots constantly crossing the globe; even more as freight ramped up. We were the only people allowed to travel anywhere. The rules were initially different everywhere, there was no consistency—wear masks, don't wear masks, stay here, don't go here. The closed loop system was supposed to be for one or two months. Initially, we had the sense that we were all in this together, but it dragged on. It was an emotional rollercoaster. The closed loop ended up lasting 19 months. If the regulations made sense and you felt it was contributing to health and safety, you put up with a lot, but you knew it was just window dressing. That was the biggest pressure. The dam broke for me once I realised Hong Kong had no metric for vaccinations that would remove the restrictions. The city went from being relatively mild by world standards, to having among the harshest restrictions in the world for aircrew by the time I finished working there in August 2022.

'We pilots are a small group of people and we're not a group that enlists a lot of public sympathy. People think we're hideously overpaid for not doing a lot of work, but a lot of people aren't aware of how global logistics works. One person said to me, "[Freight] pilots should do a two-week quarantine after each flight like everyone else." I told him that wouldn't work. There would hardly be any flights and then how would he get his stuff. He said he'd just order it online. He didn't understand that everything he ordered online had to be either flown or shipped in.'

* * *

Pilots faced the sort of pressure that can lead to psychological strains such as anxiety and PTSD, which in turn has the potential to negatively affect their ability to carry out their jobs safely (Stadler, 2022). Those working on long-haul routes had often been on a plane upwards of 18 hours when they landed in Hong Kong. Upon arrival, they were required to take a COVID-19 test and wait for about four hours on a plastic chair for the test result. In the first three days after arriving in Hong Kong, they were only permitted to leave home to get a COVID test or for essential activities. They were then required to avoid unnecessary social contact for a further 18 days and continue testing daily.

At the beginning of the pandemic, cargo flights were increased to compensate for the decrease in passenger flights and to meet the growing demand for goods. As a result, pilots who flew freight experienced a significant increase in their working hours. Many expatriate pilots working in closed-loop systems were unable to see their families for extended periods due to the quarantine requirements of both Hong Kong and their home countries, which exceeded their leave time. Currently, there is no international agreement on how quarantine measures for airline crews should be implemented, leaving individual airlines to determine all aspects of the quarantine, including accommodation, exercise, and food.

Pilots who were isolated for extended periods in hotel rooms, both during their travels and on their return, experienced a decline in morale. The pressure of working in the closed-loop system for an extended period had an accumulative effect, leading to fatigue and stress. Studies have shown that quarantine is associated with negative psychological effects, including post-traumatic stress symptoms, confusion, and anger. The longer the quarantine period, the more severe the mental health outcomes. For example, one study found that individuals quarantined for more than 10 days had significantly higher levels of posttraumatic stress symptoms than did those quarantined for less than 10 days (Hawryluck et al., 2004). Many pilots working in closed-loop systems for 18 months accumulated more than 200 days in quarantine, often without access to mental health support.

According to the Civil Aviation Department, aircrew are legally required to refrain from working if they have reason to believe they are mentally or physically unfit to fly. This places the responsibility on the individual to report unfit for duty. However, pilots were hesitant to report their mental health concerns to an aviation psychologist due to the fear of losing their medical certification, which requires them to be in good physical and mental health. They were concerned that reporting their mental health issues could have a negative impact on their future job prospects and result in them being removed from the industry (Freed, 2021).

While there is no published data specifically on the mental health of Hong Kong pilots during the pandemic, a 2022 survey of 49 commercial pilots in Asia, Europe, and North America found that 75.5 percent of pilots were stressed about their uncertain futures, antisocial working hours, and the divergence in values between pilots and management. Dr Silvia Pignata, the senior lecturer in aviation at the University of Southern Australia who led the survey, stated that the issue of work stress has been largely ignored by the aviation industry. She called for the implementation of targeted workplace measures to support pilots and reduce pilot stress (University of Southern Australia, 2022).

Pilots are perhaps the professional group best equipped to handle extended periods of quarantine. They undergo rigorous training to remain calm in emergencies and to perform tasks and checklists under pressure. If they were unable to maintain their composure in adverse conditions, they would not have completed flight training. However, they are also human, and the cumulative effect of repeated closed-loop cycles and being unable to see their families pushed many to their limits, leading to a wave of mass resignations from Cathay Pacific in 2022 (Chan & Riordan, 2022).

The current system of placing the responsibility of fitness for work solely on the pilots themselves is not sustainable. Aviation companies have a crucial role in supporting the well-being of their staff and managing sources of work-related stress. It is critical that the well-being of pilots is treated as a responsibility shared between them and their employers (Cahill et al., 2022).

There needs to be a radical rethink of the culture and processes for reporting and supporting mental well-being within the aviation industry. Ensuring that these approaches at an organisational level address both human and safety needs should be a priority, especially as Hong Kong airlines launch recruitment drives to replace the many senior pilots who resigned during the pandemic.

Strategies and Support

The advice given in the chapter on quarantine is relevant here. It is important to establish a daily routine and look after all aspects of self-care, from staying physically active, to getting enough sleep, and eating well. A Cathay Pacific pilot, who was formerly in the Swiss Army, said that the rigid discipline instilled in him from his army training helped him cope with the gruelling closed-loop system. We humans are hardwired to want certainty, so creating a routine within your own bubble will help you feel safe and secure. This will ensure that your body moves out of fight-or-flight mode and engages the parasympathetic nervous system, which allows for rest and digestion.

Make it a daily mission while in quarantine to stay in close contact with friends and family outside the industry, as well as your peers. Checking in on family members and keeping up to date with the minutiae of family life will ensure you feel connected and help you pick up where you left off when you return home. As much as possible, this contact should be either face-to-face chats on Zoom or voice calls, rather than on social media or texting. Speak to other pilots—an open sharing of experience will help you both process what you are going through. As well as venting, allow time in the conversation to share strategies for coping that you have found helpful.

This could be a good time to read up on aspects of aviation that interest you. Sharing that knowledge with friends in the industry can deepen your personal connections as well as reinforce your learning.

If you have time on your hands, you might consider writing a journal. You could use your journal to set out goals or healthy habits that you want to work towards, or as an opportunity to process what you are going through. Journaling has been shown to be a great way of reducing stress and focusing on the things that aren't working for you. Even starting with something as simple as spending a few minutes a day writing down five things you are grateful for can boost your mental well-being and help shift your focus from a negative mindset to a positive one.

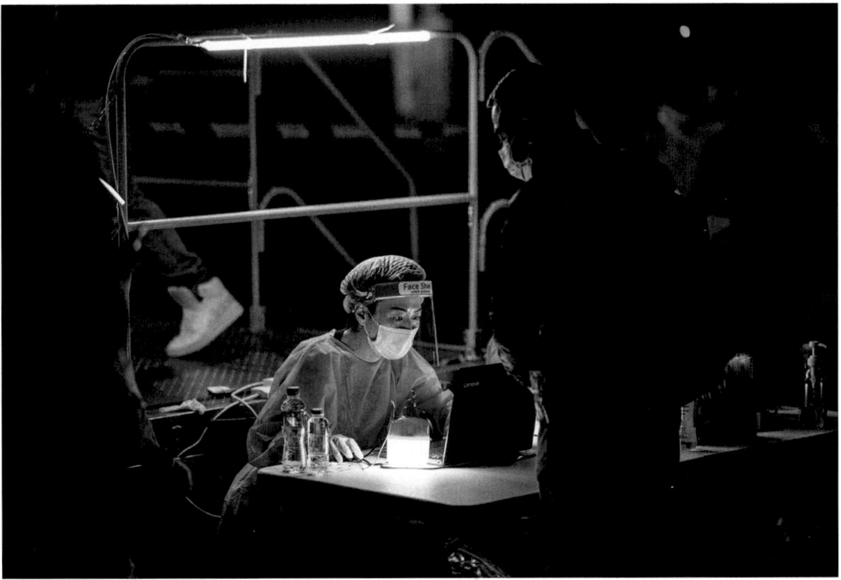

A resident registered for a mandatory COVID-19 test on January 22, 2021 in the Jordan area of the Yau Tsim Mong district, a densely populated area which saw a spike in coronavirus cases over the winter. Photo by Anthony Wallace © AFP.

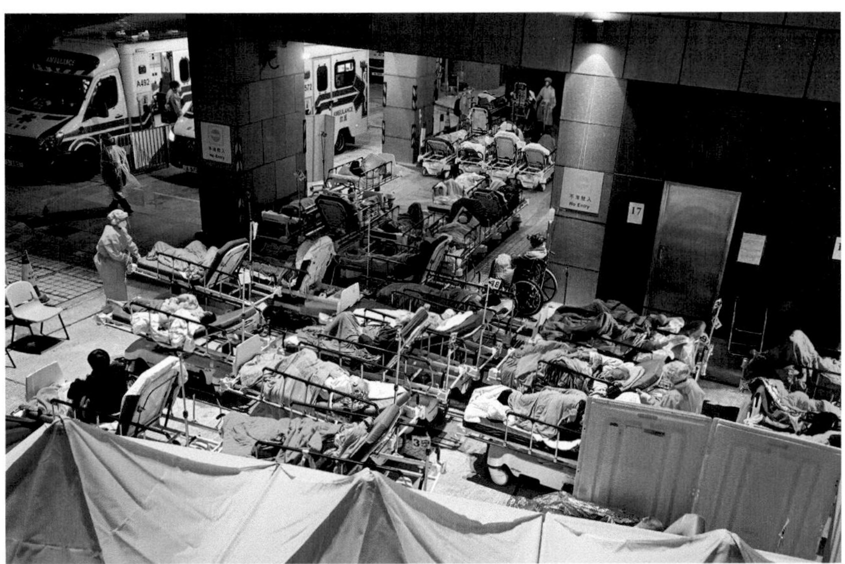

People lay in hospital beds outside the Caritas Medical Centre on February 16, 2022 as hospitals were overwhelmed by the deadly 'fifth wave', the darkest period of Hong Kong's COVID-19 pandemic. Photo by Peter Parks © AFP.

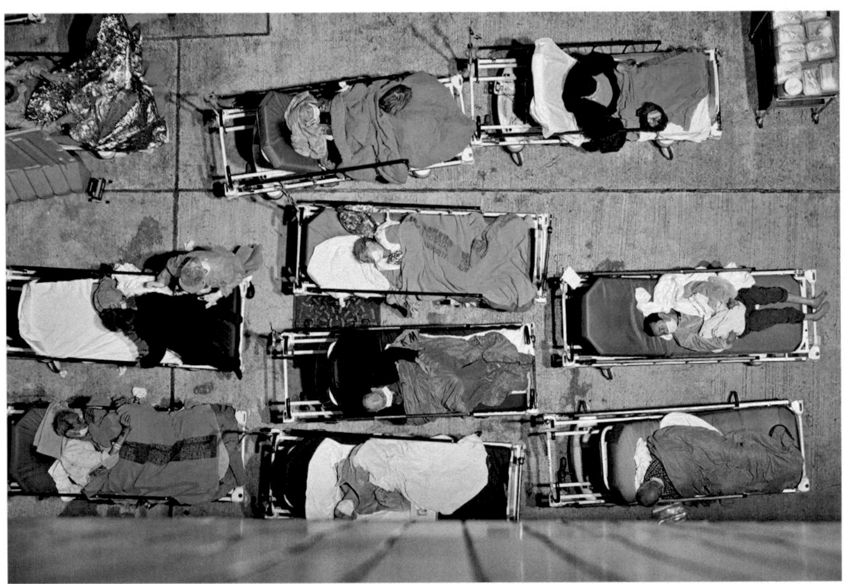

COVID-19 patients were forced to wait outside Hong Kong's public hospitals in the cold in February 2022 for hours before admission. Once inside, some had to stay in corridors or even bathrooms until a bed was vacated for them. Photo by Peter Parks © AFP.

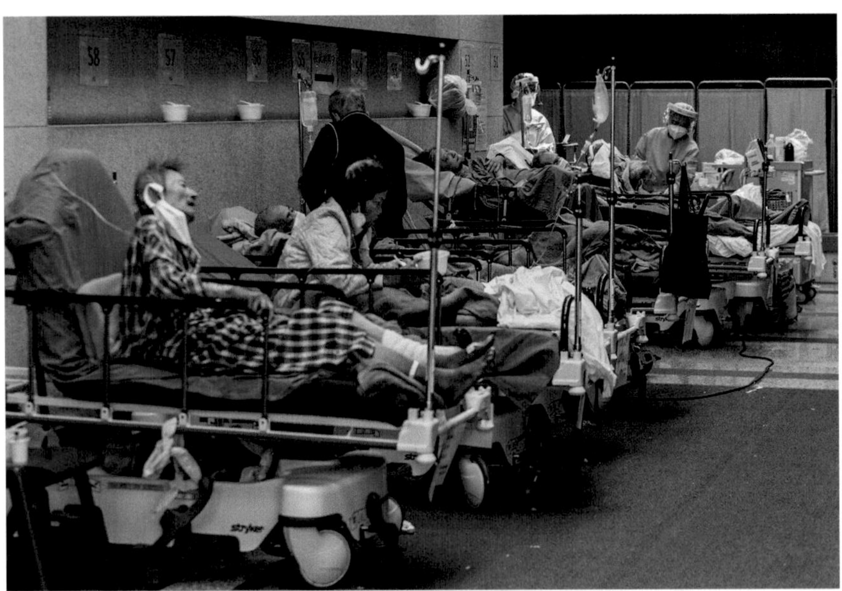

Health workers wearing PPE treated patients in a holding area next to the accident and emergency department of Princess Margaret hospital in Hong Kong on March 11, 2022 as the city faced its worst-ever COVID-19 outbreak. Photo by Dale de la Rey © AFP.

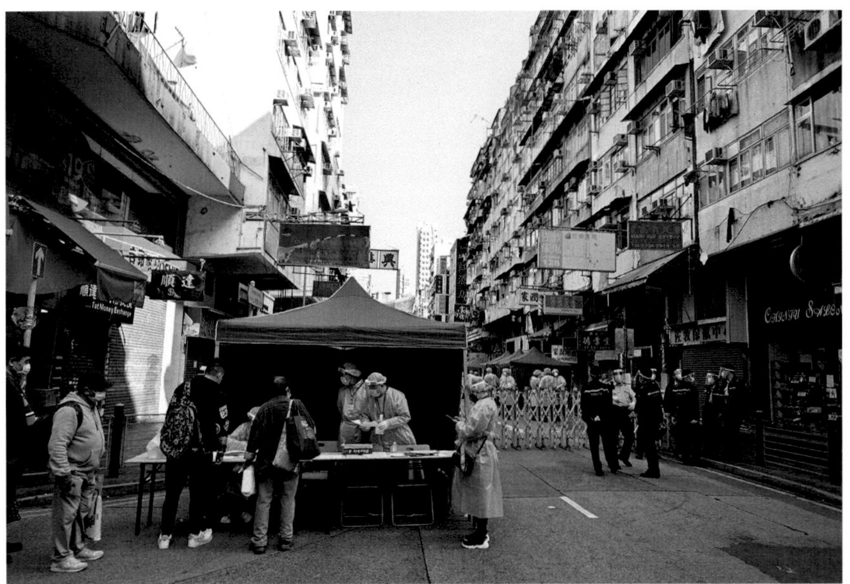

The lockdown of Jordan—an area known for its old and subdivided dwellings, and home to many poor and elderly residents—impacted about 10,000 residents. Photo by Peter Parks © AFP.

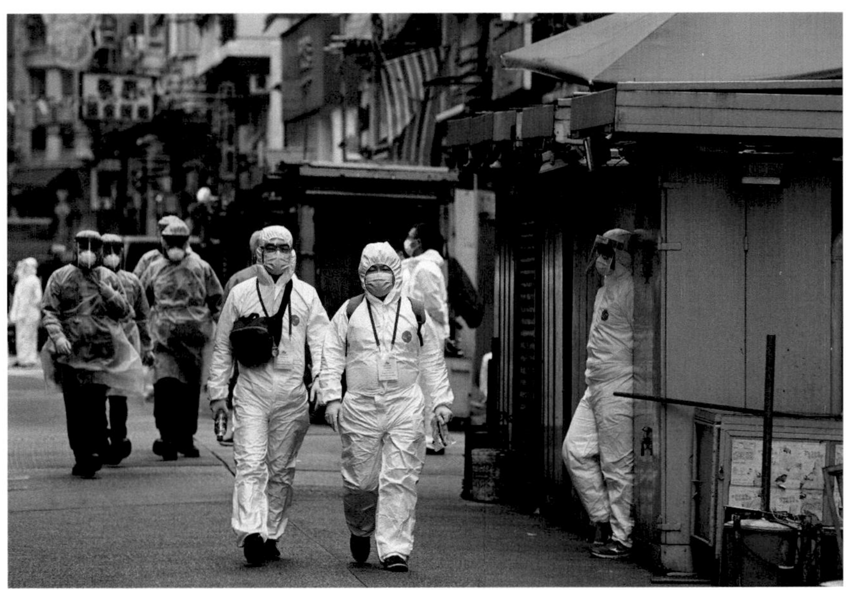

Health workers clad in white hazmat suits walked along a street as authorities continued testing for the second day in Jordan on January 24, 2021. Thousands of residents were ordered to stay in their homes for the city's first COVID-19 lockdown. Photo by Peter Parks © AFP.

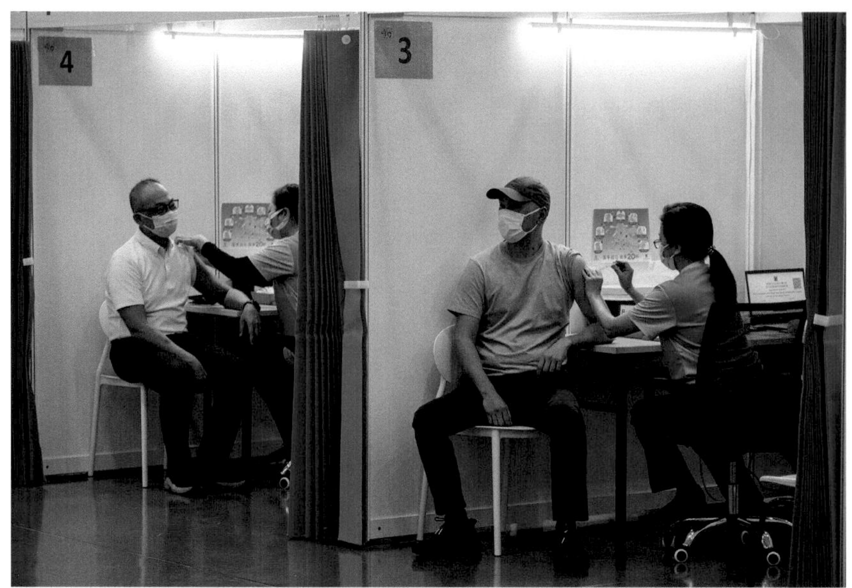

Hong Kong residents received a dose of China's Sinovac COVID-19 coronavirus vaccine at a community vaccination centre. They were given the option to choose between Sinovac and Pfizer/BioNTech vaccines. Photo by Paul Yeung / POOL / © AFP.

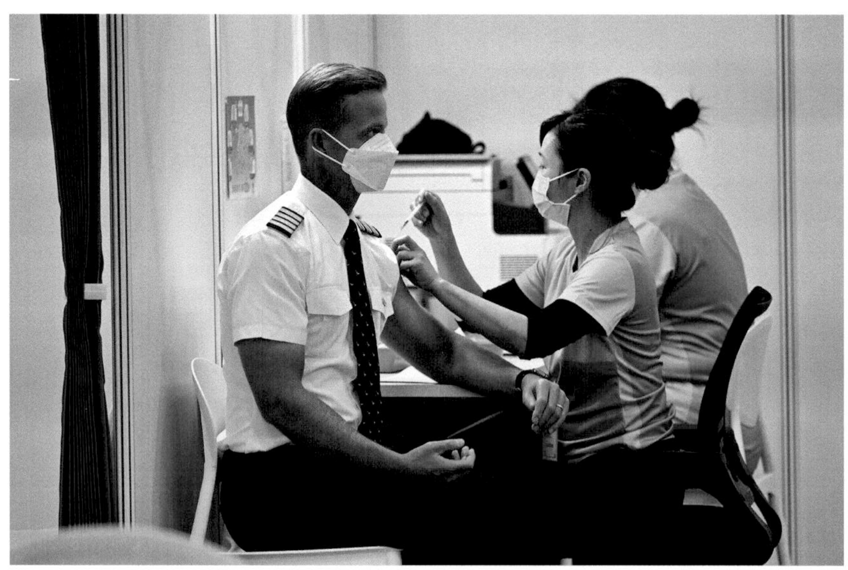

A Cathay Pacific pilot received China's Sinovac COVID-19 coronavirus vaccine at a community vaccination centre in February 2021, the month in which the airline began running 'closed loop' rosters in order to staff flights from countries such as the UK and US that were deemed 'high risk'. Photo by Peter Parks and Peter Parks / POOL / © AFP.

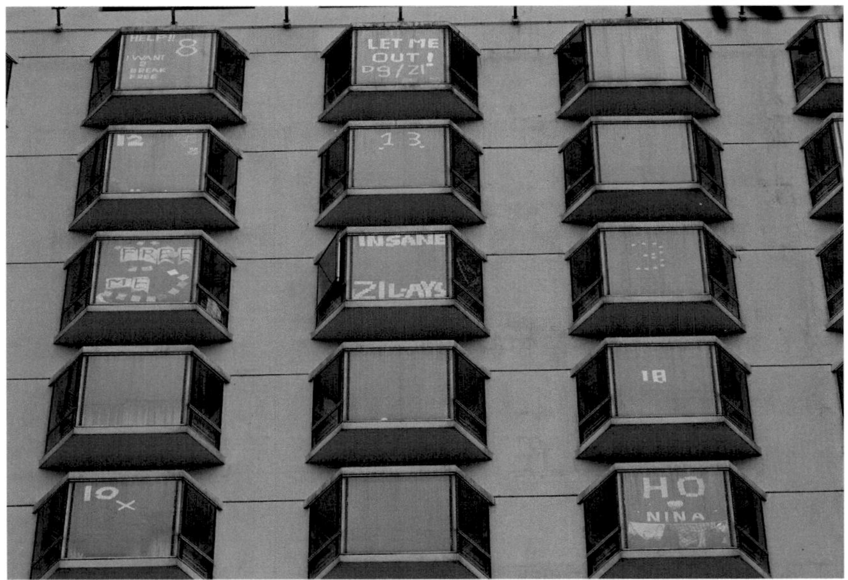

Hong Kong's three-week hotel quarantine was one of the longest COVID-19 quarantines in the world. At some hotels, quarantined guests posted messages in the window counting down the days of their incarceration. Photo by Peter Parks © AFP.

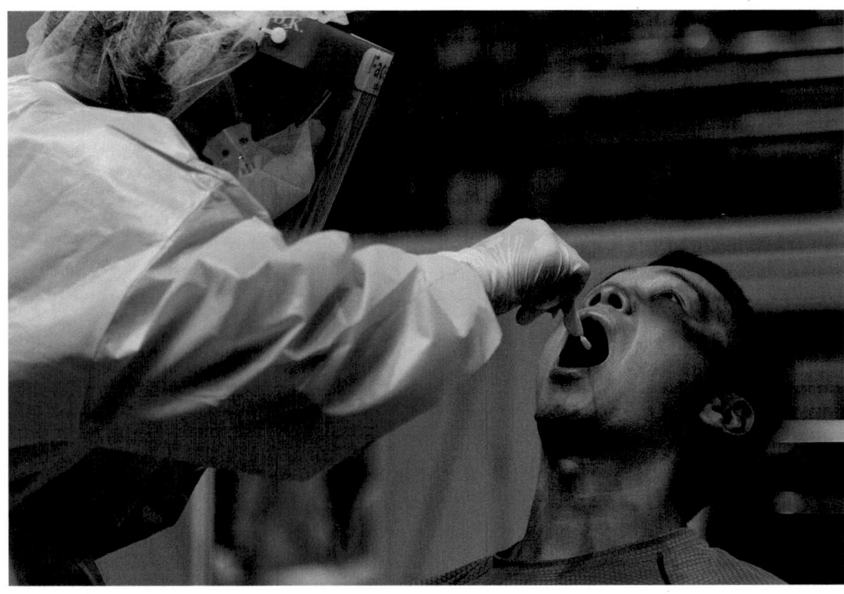

A swab sample was collected from a man by a medical worker at a makeshift testing site for COVID-19 infections at Queen Elizabeth Stadium on September 1, 2020, the day Hong Kong launched a mass coronavirus testing scheme. Photo by Anthony Kwan / POOL / ©AFP.

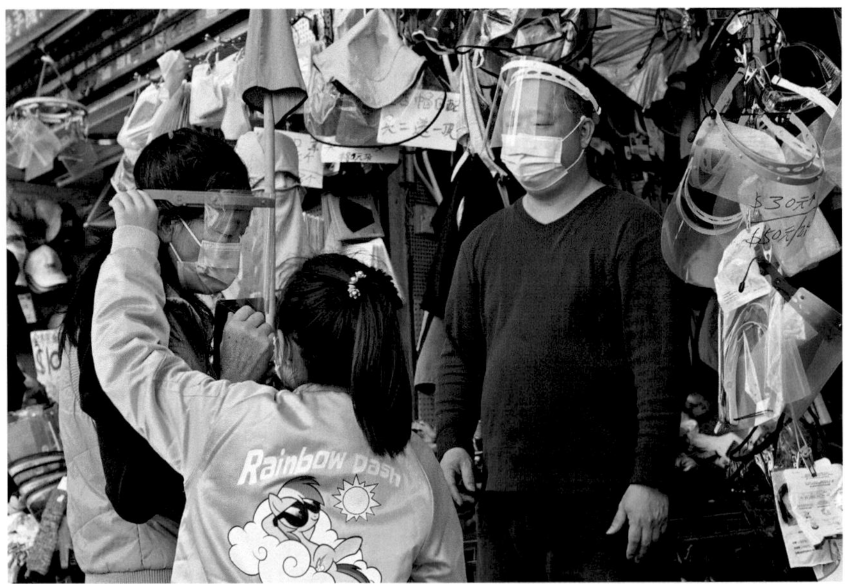

A woman tried on a face shield to protect against COVID-19 in February 2022. The prolonged wearing of face masks meant that children grew up without being able to see the expressions of those around them, limiting their ability to read social cues and stunting their social development. Photo by Peter Parks © AFP.

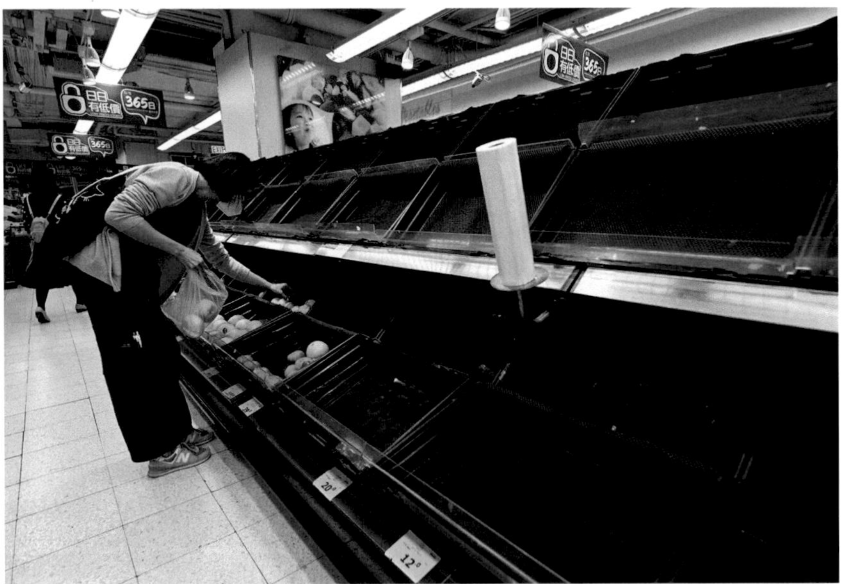

Mixed messages from authorities about a planned lockdown and mass testing of the city's population in March 2022 led to a frenzied stripping of supermarket shelves and sending food prices soaring. Photo by Peter Parks © AFP.

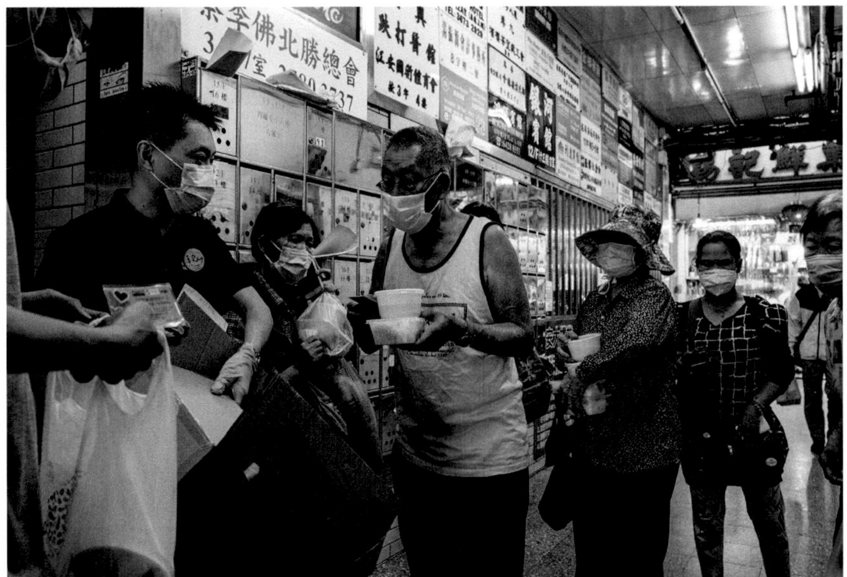

People queued up in Yau Ma Tei to receive free meal boxes from Gingko House, a social enterprise devoted to promoting elderly employment in catering services. Photo by Anthony Wallace © AFP.

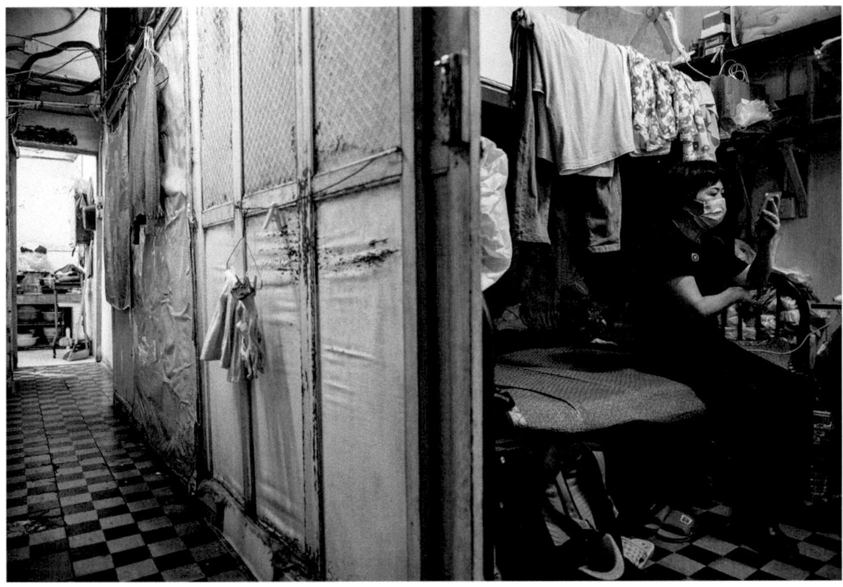

This walk-up flat in the New Territories is subdivided into six cubicles. Wong Mei-ying, 70, shares a 50-square-foot living space with her son. The corridor leads to a communal kitchen and bathroom. Crowded living conditions in subdivided flats made social distancing especially challenging. Photo by Anthony Wallace © AFP.

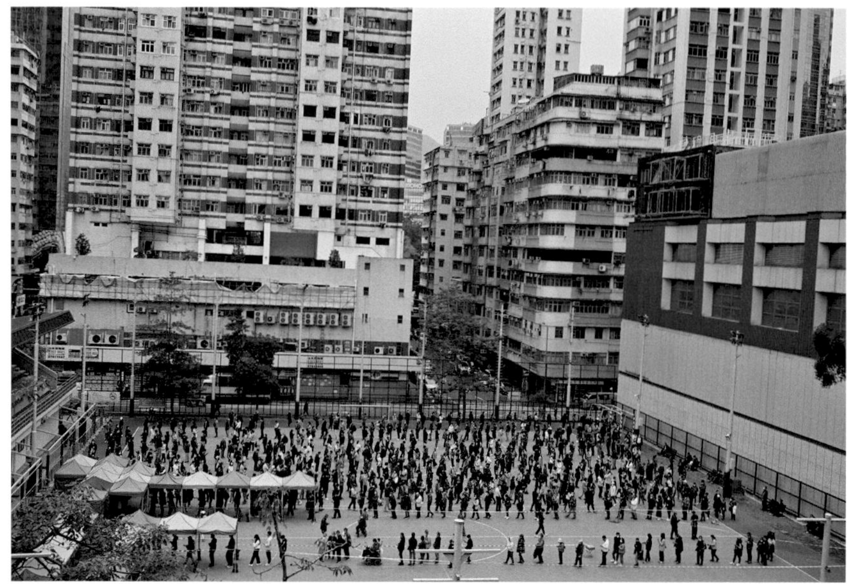

People queued at a mobile specimen collection station for COVID-19 testing in Hong Kong's Mong Kok district on February 10, 2022 as authorities scrambled to ramp up testing capacity following a record high number of new infections. Photo by Peter Parks © AFP.

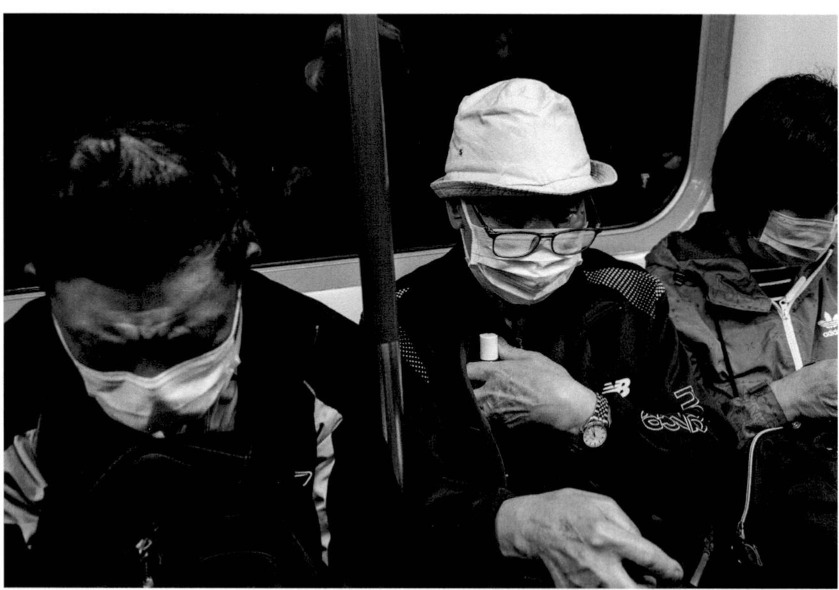

Passengers wore face masks on a Mass Transit Railway (MTR) train in Hong Kong in March 2020. The mask mandate was lifted on March 1, 2023, but many people continued to wear face masks in public. Photo by Anthony Wallace © AFP.

9

Migrant Workers

Hong Kong is home to one of the highest densities of foreign domestic workers in the world, about 400,000 individuals mostly from the Philippines and Indonesia. These workers play a crucial role in Hong Kong's economy by freeing up women from domestic duties and allowing them to join the workforce. More than 90 percent of these workers are women, and many are wives and mothers. The pandemic made it difficult for these workers to see their families, and many were worried about losing their job and not being able to support their loved ones back home, who depend on them financially.

In Hong Kong, foreign domestic workers are required by law to live in their employer's home. As flats in the city are small, it is common for these workers to be forced to share a room with a child or older people or to sleep in the living room, kitchen, or even toilet (Carnay, 2017). The pandemic made things worse for these workers, as school closures and working from home led to homes being full, further eroding the little free time and space they had.

Tasked with keeping their employer's home clean, these women were frontline workers in fighting the virus. Yet during the pandemic they were often portrayed as people spreading the virus (Chau, 2023). According to a 2020 study by the Chinese University of Hong Kong, migrant domestic workers in Hong Kong had worse self-rated mental health than did the general adult Hong Kong population, due to their financial circumstances, living conditions, work pressure, negative job-related experiences, and socio-demographic characteristics (Chung & Mak, 2020).

***Catalina** has been working as a domestic helper in Hong Kong for 23 years. During the pandemic, she faced a challenging period when three sets of employers left Hong Kong within the span of just three years. The financial pressure and stress of finding new employment, compounded by testing positive for COVID-19 twice, led her into a state of depression. However, with the support of free counselling provided by a non-governmental organisation, the 50-year-old has emerged from this difficult time stronger and more resilient.*

'In 2020, my employer left Hong Kong because of COVID, so I needed to find another employer. After one year with my new employer, they also left because of the situation in Hong Kong. I got COVID for the first time in 2021; it was a bad year. Moving jobs three times in three years was stressful. In February 2022, my new employer was pregnant and expecting a baby in three weeks when I got COVID again. I couldn't stay at my employer's house because I didn't want to infect them, and I couldn't go to hospital because then she wouldn't be able to deliver her baby at the hospital. If the hospital knew there was a COVID-positive person in the same house they wouldn't have let her enter. So, I stayed at a boarding house. I was in a small room by myself because I didn't want anyone to catch the virus. I just stayed in that room waiting for whatever help I could get.

It was difficult. When I recovered from COVID, I wasn't feeling like my old self.

'My employer had her baby. A baby is therapeutic, and although work was busy the baby gave me a lot of happiness. Then when the baby was three months old, my employers went away for two months. The house was quiet; there was nothing to do. It was a time when there were heavy restrictions about gatherings. I was lonely and alone. All the accumulated stress and everything suddenly went boom. It was a perfect storm, a super typhoon. I felt so alone. There was fear. I didn't go out; I just wanted to lie down. I felt so weak and tired and wanted to sleep all day and night. I didn't want to bathe. I didn't feel hungry. One day I realised I hadn't eaten for a day and went to the fridge. It was empty. I left the flat and the security guard downstairs said I hadn't been out for two weeks. He didn't know there was anyone in the flat.

'That was when I realised I had to do something. I thought if I didn't ask for help, I might hurt myself, but I hadn't reached that point yet. I called my friends and told them I was very lonely. One of them put me in touch with a counsellor in the Philippines. She charged 750 pesos for a one-hour meeting on Zoom. The trouble was she was very busy, and it was hard to get another appointment. Although it wasn't that expensive, it was still money I couldn't afford. I called my friend Rodelia. She'd had depression in the past and we'd talked about it. Rodelia called the NGO HELP for Domestic Workers, and they put me in touch with a counsellor called Heda.

'Heda is also Filipino, and she helped me a lot. Speaking to her in my own language, it made it so much easier to open up. Because we have a shared culture, she understood what to ask to get me to open up. She really listened to me and I felt that she understood what I was feeling. She didn't force me to talk. I felt that I was opening up because I wanted to. Talking about things made me feel so much better. I had a session with her every week for two months, and she texted me in between. It felt good to have someone checking in on me.

'I also learned skills to help myself, like EFT [Emotional Freedom Techniques]. Now when I feel anxious, I use tapping to help myself. I also do it with friends when they are stressed. I learned breathing techniques to calm myself and I enjoy yoga nidra. When the yoga teacher, Myriam Bartu, offers free online sessions, she tells me, and I join. After my depression, I started volunteering and doing migrant initiatives. For me, my depression was a turning point where I rediscovered my strength. One of my friends thinks of depression as a way to find out your deeper person. I definitely changed through that dark time and I am stronger now.

'In the migrant worker community, there is a lot of stigma about mental health. There is a thinking that if you ask for help you are weak, which means that many people don't ask for help when they need it. There is a culture in the Philippines that makes people afraid to tell their story. You are afraid that people will talk about you and that what you say will go back to the Philippines. Many of my friends don't tell their problems to their family. We try to pretend that we are superhuman, but in reality we are not.

'Many migrant workers are not aware that there are NGOs that can help you. They don't know you can get free counselling if you need it. In the Bible it says, "Ask and you will receive". But many people don't ask, so they don't get help. Helping yourself should start with you; you have to open up. I want to share my story; I want to tell people to not be afraid to seek help. When you talk, choose who you open up to wisely. Speak to trusted friends, NGOs, or counsellors.

'I think that people's mental health is getting worse after COVID. During COVID we were just going and going. We were in fight-or-flight mode and we kept fighting. Then when the body is able to rest, it goes "boom!" It was like my experience. I was so stressed and worried, but I kept going and kept busy. When my employers went away and I had a rest and nothing to do, that was when my depression came out. This is what I see happening in Hong Kong; people's mental health is getting worse.'

***Miriam** (not her real name), a 36-year-old domestic helper from Luzon in the Philippines, had been working for a family of four in North Point for a decade. She had helped raise their two daughters and had grown accustomed to the stable world she knew. However, when her employer lost his job during the pandemic, her world imploded, and she hit rock bottom.*

'After so many years looking after the two girls, I was very close to them and felt like a second mother. When COVID started, they were at university and staying in a dorm on campus. I was very afraid of COVID and was careful to make sure I did not get it. I stayed at home most of the time and didn't see my friends much. I wanted to keep my employers safe.

'In June 2022, my employer lost his job. He told me they needed to cut some expenses and could not afford to pay my salary, so they terminated my contract. They gave me one month notice and a long-service payment. My employer's wife knows the daughters are close to me. She didn't want them to know that I was terminated. She said it would upset them, so she told them that I was going to move back to the Philippines. My employer was crying when she asked me not to tell her daughters. I'd been with the family for so many years and then I was terminated. It was hurtful; they felt like family.

'They let me stay for one week while I looked for another job, but after a week I had to leave because they'd told the daughters that I was getting a flight to the Philippines. I felt so stressed. If I went to a boarding house, I'd need to pay to stay there and would need to pay for my food. I have a little savings, but not enough. I was so worried and devastated.

'A friend at church told me about MercyHK and said they had a shelter and that the food is free. I felt so relieved because before that I didn't know where I was going to sleep. I didn't know there was this kind of thing in Hong Kong. Before that I didn't even know what "NGO" means. Even though I was terminated, I felt so lucky that I had found a place to stay. The agency found me another employer in Yuen Long, but I needed to wait a week for my visa. I shared the hostel with two girls. After a week, I got my visa. The day that I was supposed to meet my new employer, I found out that one of the girls in the hostel had COVID. The other girl and I did a rapid test, and we were both also positive. Oh my god, I was so worried that my new employer would terminate me. I felt ashamed about getting COVID. I told the agency and they told the new employer.

'I know that employers don't like it if you get COVID, so I was very worried. I was stressed, sad, devastated—I didn't know what was going to happen.

'I reported to the government that I was positive in the morning, and they told me I needed to go to Penny's Bay. I'd heard the stories about Penny's Bay, so I was nervous. The shuttle bus came to collect me at 1 am. The bus picked up a few more people, and we arrived at the quarantine centre at about 3 am. It was very dark, and I didn't know what was going to happen. People in hazmat suits showed me to a room. When I was inside the room, they opened the window and spoke to me through the window and told me the rules and how to order food on the app.

'It made me feel uncomfortable knowing that I couldn't go out of the room, but I got used to it after a few days. The food was ok. I could choose what I wanted to eat, and they brought it. The bed was uncomfortable—the mattress was very thin and covered in plastic which made a crunchy sound when I moved. I'd had three vaccinations, so my symptoms were mild.

'I was so worried about my employer and whether my contract would be terminated. Would I have a job? There was so much on my mind that I couldn't sleep well. I spent a lot of time praying and watching TV. I spoke to my family in Luzon almost every hour when I was in quarantine. They were very worried for me.

'After a week, I did a PCR test and they let me go back to the shelter. I got the result of the PCR test when I was in the shelter. I was still positive. The agency told me to wait a few more days until I was fully recovered. After three days I got another PCR test at a community centre and that one showed I was now negative. I was so happy. Luckily my employer waited for me and I went to her house in Yuen Long. On my first day, she didn't give me a lot of work to do. She was nice. Later, I learned that she'd had COVID. She understood it wasn't my fault I got COVID and didn't blame me.'

***Lydia**, a 35-year-old single mother from the Philippines, has been working as a domestic helper in Hong Kong for 10 years. She sends her salary back home to pay for her sons' education. Although she's usually resilient, a series of unfortunate events during the pandemic left her feeling isolated and chipped away at her mental health.*

'I started working for my employer at the end of 2020. I did the cleaning and cooking and looked after their child. My employer was very worried about COVID. They thought that if I went out of the house and had a gathering with my friends, I might get COVID and bring it back to the family. Sometimes they sent me to clean my employer's mother's house. Sunday is my day off, but ma'am and sir wanted to go out and needed someone to look after their child, so they paid me to work on Sundays.

'My mother is also a domestic helper in Hong Kong, but I couldn't see her. And I couldn't see my friends or go to church. I started to feel very lonely. The only people I saw were my employers. In 2021, after I was with the family for six months, I got COVID. My employer didn't want me to stay with them, so they sent me to their mother's house, which was empty. They gave me food and medicine and told me to stay in the flat and not go outside. I was there for three weeks. It felt like a very long time to be alone. After three weeks, I went back to my employer. As soon as I got back, they terminated my contract. They said they had financial problems because of COVID-19.

'I was so sad because I had no work and no place to live. My mother knows a priest, and I went to speak to the father. He told me about a shelter where I could stay. I stayed in the hostel for one month and waited to get another job. It was not easy to find another employer and make an adjustment to another family. Because I was only working for my employer for six months it made it difficult to get another job. People might ask, "Why were you only there six months? What did you do wrong?"

'I found another employer in Tai Koo Shing, but they were not good. I had to start work at 6 am and work non-stop until 10 pm. They gave me no rest. They didn't give me enough food, so I was hungry most of the time. I was so unhappy; I didn't know what to do and cried a lot. I couldn't control my emotions. I've never cried like that. I wasn't myself. I have two sons in the Philippines; one is 10 years old and the other is 18. I missed them but I didn't want to call them because I didn't want them to hear me crying.

'After one month, I left. I went back to the shelter for two weeks and then to the Philippines. I wanted to see my sons and rest and recover. After some months in the Philippines, a friend recommended me to an employer. I took the job. I need to earn money to pay for my sons' school, and later I want them to go to college. Now that things are more stable, I have Sundays off and can meet my friends.'

***Gloria** (not her real name), a 55-year-old domestic helper from the Philippines, has been working for her employers for 16 years and helped raise their two children. She considers them to be fair and reasonable employers but found the pandemic very stressful.*

'When we were all together at home, all five of us in the flat, my world was too small. I couldn't really move. My stress at that time was 10/10. Before, I used to move around the house doing the cleaning, and after that I could exercise and move easily, but with so many people studying and working in the house I had to be quiet. Normally I don't spend so much time with them, but with ma'am always there and looking at me, it was very stressful. After eating, I just sat down, and my tummy got so heavy and I got fat. I felt bored, so I ate more. Sometimes I found it quite hard to get to sleep. Some domestic helpers didn't want to take the vaccine, and some of my friends say it's a poison, but for me it was okay. I've had three vaccinations.

'My ma'am let me have my day off. I have been working in Hong Kong 20 years, and I always spend my Sundays doing service at the church, but during the pandemic the service was cancelled. Instead, I met my church friends in Central. Going out, you had to wear a mask, which I found uncomfortable. It was hard to breathe. Even if you are wearing a mask and you cough just a little, Chinese people stare at you and their eyes get really big. You could burp and fart and they didn't notice, but if you coughed, they really stared at you.

'The police were very aggressive towards us. They kept coming up to us, making sure we were wearing a mask, reminding us to keep our distance and checking to see we were no more than four in our group. When I was outside, I was always on the alert. "Be careful, the police are coming." It was stressful, and I worried about the people who were caught by the police.

'Because the police were so aggressive, I decided to avoid town on my day off and started to go on hikes. Sometimes the police were waiting for us on the hiking trails. They were near the entrance to Lion Rock Country Park. It made me very anxious when the police stared at us, so we started going to remote places where there was less chance the police would be waiting for us.

'For me, hiking was the blessing of the pandemic. I felt like a bird let out of its cage. During the pandemic, I discovered lots of good places in Hong Kong. On my day off, I hiked around Lantau Island, and one time I even climbed the highest mountain in Hong Kong, Tai Mo Shan. I'm thankful to the pandemic for that.

'My employer is a lawyer. She told me, "I can't make you stay home on your day off, but remember, if the police catch you for not wearing a mask or something, they will fine you." When the police increased the fine from HK$5,000 to HK$10,000 I was very worried. That is a huge amount of money. If I got fined HK$10,000 it would be the worst. Sometimes, when my employer reminded me about the fine, I chose to stay at home and do Bible study online with my friends from the church.

'I was very worried about my family in the Philippines, especially my mother. I haven't been home for five years. My family are stressed. They thought that the COVID situation in Hong Kong was very dangerous, especially when they found out that domestic workers were not being allowed into hospital and had to wait outside. Some helpers were terminated by their employers when they got the virus. That was really terrible. What kind of employer does that? My family said to me, "Take care of yourself." I said, "Don't worry about me; I go hiking in the high mountains. I feel like a bird on the top of the mountain. I have a healthy place during my holiday, so don't worry about me."

'In December [2021], my employer's eldest daughter got COVID. Oh my god, I went everywhere in Hong Kong and never got COVID and then I got it at home. We all got COVID. My employer reported to the government that we are sick. It was a stressful time for me. I felt quite sick, but even though I was a COVID patient, I was also taking care of COVID patients. My employer wouldn't let me open the back door to take out the rubbish. I tied up the rubbish in plastic bags and after one week there was a big pile of bags in the kitchen. It was disgusting; I hated it. I thought my employer was really OA [over acting], but she said she was worried the police would catch me if I opened the door to take the rubbish out. Looking after them when I had COVID was the hardest part of the pandemic.'

* * *

During the pandemic, foreign domestic workers in Hong Kong were faced with an increased workload. In addition to their usual duties, they had to sanitise and sterilise their employer's home, look after young children during the school closures, take care of the elderly, who were most vulnerable to the virus, and queue for a long time to buy daily essentials. All this was done under the close scrutiny of their employer, who was now working from home. There are no legal regulations on the maximum working hours of foreign domestic workers in Hong Kong, which makes them vulnerable to exploitation. This caused many of them to feel stressed, tired, exhausted, and burnt out (Lui et al., 2021).

Concern over job security was a major stressor for many workers, especially because many of them are the breadwinners for their families back home. Within their social groups, many had heard stories of friends who had lost their job for COVID-related reasons or because their employer had lost their job and could no longer afford to pay them. If they were made redundant, they were obliged by law to find another job within two weeks or pay for a visa extension.

Foreign domestic workers are entitled to one day off a week, usually on a Sunday. However, during the pandemic they received pressure from both their employers and the government to stay home on their rest day. In 2020, the government issued no fewer than 15 press releases on this issue. The day off on a Sunday represents not just a chance to physically separate themselves from their workplace but also to see their friends. Social connections are one of the most important means of safeguarding mental health for this vulnerable group. They offer an opportunity for emotional support and stress release. Given that family is overseas, connecting with peers who share common beliefs, culture, and experiences is critical for stress coping and mental health support.

The Hong Kong government initially imposed a fine of HK$2,000 for breaching anti-pandemic rules. The fine was later raised to HK$10,000 for violations that included not wearing a face mask, gathering in groups, and missing mandatory COVID-19 tests. Many migrant domestic workers fell afoul of the restrictions, especially those arriving in Hong Kong, who were confused by the ever-changing testing requirements. Migrant workers' minimum monthly salary is HK$4,730, so a HK$10,000 penalty was more than two months' salary. Police officers were deployed to enforce social-distancing rules in areas where domestic workers tend to gather during their day off, such as parks and pavements.

Financial woes were a huge source of anxiety for many. The pandemic intensified the economic strain in their home country, putting even more pressure on foreign domestic workers, who are often the primary breadwinners for their families. According to a survey conducted by HelperChoice (2022), 40 percent of 546 domestic helpers felt stressed because of their financial situation. Nearly 28 percent had to send more money home than before, while almost 20 percent saw their expenses rise. But the toll wasn't just financial. Over half the workers surveyed reported sleeping only four to six hours a night, well below the minimum seven hours recommended. The effects of insufficient sleep are alarming, leading to reduced physical strength, a weakened immune system, and increased levels of anxiety.

In early 2022, foreign domestic workers in the city faced an unprecedented crisis during the fifth wave of COVID-19. Although quarantine in a government facility was mandatory at the time, the camps were overwhelmed by the sheer number of COVID cases, and many people recovered at home before a space became available in an official camp. Some domestic workers who contracted the virus were told by their employers they couldn't live with them while they were COVID positive even though legally their employer was obliged to house them for the duration of their contract. This left them homeless. The shocking situation made international headlines and prompted local charities to step in to provide shelter. The

NGO HELP for Domestic Workers helped more than 800 domestic workers over two months during the fifth wave (Chau, 2023).

As the pandemic evolved, confusion and uncertainty spread among foreign domestic workers. Many struggled to understand information released in the media, and with fake news rampant on social media, concerns arose about their ability to accurately assess information related to communicable diseases (Ho & Smith, 2020). A study of Filipina domestic workers found that language and cultural barriers must be addressed to ensure that these workers can understand and follow public health recommendations (Yeung et al., 2020).

Migrant domestic workers are often left to fend for themselves when it comes to mental health. The lack of education and support in this area is a glaring omission that demands attention. This is a group of people who often find solace in the company of their peers. Far from their families, they form tight bonds with those they share a culture and background with. In fact, a 2020 study revealed that only 22 percent turn to NGOs for help in times of distress, preferring instead to rely on their own close-knit community (Uplifters, 2020). By nurturing these social networks, we can support the mental well-being of these workers. One promising approach is para-professional peer support training, which has been shown to be both effective and culturally sensitive. By expanding such programmes, we can empower women and promote mental health awareness within the already established support networks (Ho et al., 2022).

As Hong Kong braces for an ageing population, the demand for migrant domestic workers is expected to surge to 600,000 by 2031. But with China poised to open its labour market and offer higher wages, Hong Kong may struggle to compete (Wong, 2021). The COVID-19 pandemic has already taken a toll on migrant workers in

Hong Kong, and if their grievances are not addressed, they may seek opportunities elsewhere.

Strategies and Support

Stress and anxiety are two sides of the same coin, but they're not quite the same thing. Stress is often caused by external pressures that we struggle to handle, while anxiety can be more elusive: It's often focused on worries or fears about things that could threaten us, as well as anxiety about the anxiety itself. While stress can be easier to pinpoint and manage, anxiety can be more difficult to work out.

Stress and anxiety are both natural emotions, especially during times of uncertainty like a pandemic. But when these feelings persist for a long time or start to affect our daily lives, it's important to address them. Trying to ignore or suppress uncomfortable feelings may feel like the brave thing to do, but it only makes them stronger. Instead, we should stop struggling against them and acknowledge and accept them: This can help us release their grip on us.

Managing stress, anxiety, and other powerful emotion can be challenging, but this four-step process can help:

- NOTICE / Feel what is happening inside your body. Is your heart racing? Are your shoulders tight? Our bodies have automatic warning systems designed to keep us safe, but they are just warnings and don't always mean we are in danger. So, begin by noticing the physical sensations in your body.
- NAME / Give the emotion that you are feeling a name. Are you angry? Sad? Worried? By labelling what we are feeling, we better understand what is happening.

- ACCEPT / Sit non-judgmentally with what you are feeling and accept it without trying to control it. Accepting a negative emotion doesn't mean you have to accept the situation that leads to that emotion.
- NAVIGATE / Decide what would be a useful way to react. It can be useful to consider whether this happened before. How did you respond in the past? Did it teach you a lesson about how to respond in the future? Is there a friend you can talk to about how you are feeling? Do you need to ask for help?

During a pandemic, the opportunities to gather are restricted, which can lead to isolation and feelings of hopelessness and helplessness. Although mental health education, support, and resources for domestic workers in Hong Kong are limited, there are established organisations and community groups dedicated to offering advice and emergency support for migrant workers. As long as you have a phone or an internet connection, you can connect to these groups and request help. You are never alone.

Christian Action has two service centres (Mong Kok and Sheung Shui) that offer psychological counselling and consultation, emergency shelter, rights-based and critical consultation services, education workshops, and recreational activities.

http://christian-action.org.hk/en/hong-kong/humanitarian-social-services/migrant-domestic-workers
Contact: +852 5269 7332

HELP for Domestic Workers is a non-profit organisation that offers advice and assistance, awareness and education, and empowerment and peer support for migrant domestic workers. HELP can provide advice on legal questions, case counselling, education on rights and responsibilities, emergency shelter, and mental well-being support.

http://helpfordomesticworkers.org
Contact: +852 2523 4020 / +852 5936 3780
WhatsApp (English and Filipino): +852 5936 3780

Bethune House provides temporary accommodation, food, medical support, and legal help for migrant women workers. Every week, six or seven migrants in distress approach the centre for support and usually stay in the shelter for two weeks to two months.

http://bethunehouse.org
Contact: +852 2721 3119

PathFinders is a charity dedicated to supporting the children born to migrant mothers. If you are a migrant worker who has become pregnant or given birth to a child in Hong Kong, call the hotline for support. This includes workers who have overstayed their visa.

Website: www.pathfinders.org.hk
Hotline for migrant workers: +852 5190 4886

10

Uncertainty

Is it safe to be vaccinated? What will happen if I get COVID? Will I be sent to Penny's Bay Quarantine Centre? When will schools reopen? When will the travel ban be lifted? Will I be separated from my child? When will quarantine end? Will I lose my job? So much about the pandemic was unexpected and unknown, and this stoked an overriding sense of uncertainty, which fuelled anxiety. For many people, all the unanswered questions and inability to plan ahead chipped away at their resilience and undermined their mental health. The fear of the unknown and the constant barrage of news about the virus left many feeling overwhelmed and helpless.

***Winnie Cheung** (not her real name) is in her early 40s and works in the wellness industry. She found herself overwhelmed by the constant stream of COVID-19 news. For two years, she spent two to three hours a day gathering information and cross-checking conflicting reports, leaving her feeling anxious. The alarming vaccine stories she read in the local press and on social media caused her to delay getting vaccinated* *until it became mandatory for her to continue going to work and dining at restaurants.*

'I don't trust medication that is very new; it means they haven't had enough time to do proper research on it. A friend working in the medical industry in the US told me that a lot of vaccines and medications were being offered for free or at low prices to Asia in exchange for data and to find out if they were any good. I didn't want to be a guinea pig. Also, I have a vagus nerve issue and an irregular heartbeat, which means I faint easily, so I'm wary about what I put in my body.

'I followed the news closely on the local TV, mostly TVB, and some websites. In the beginning, the Chinese news kept changing the story; they would say one thing and then another. First of all, they tried to push people to take vaccines and said if you don't do it you will die. Then they said if you are a certain age take this one, if you are another age that one, and they kept changing the advice. It made me feel anxious. There were also stories about people who died after having the vaccine. They said there was no evidence that the death was related to the vaccine, but of course it makes you wonder. I was always wondering who was telling the lie. The story was always shifting, and I started to feel the news was playing tricks with the numbers. I read a paper written by a doctor in the US, and although I couldn't understand everything he said, it made me feel that Pfizer was really new and there were a lot of unknowns.

'Every day I checked the news to see if there were any quarantine buildings near my place or my parents' home. If I found one of the affected buildings was near them, I'd tell them to stay away and not to go to the market near there. Checking the news and updates online and checking with friends took a lot of time and was very stressful. I always wanted to double-check that what I was reading was correct.

When my mum caught COVID, I noticed that my parents' building was not on the list, which made me realise the system wasn't accurate. If we were told there were 1,000 cases, I guessed it was really a lot more than that.

'There were COVID press conferences every day. The journalists kept asking questions, and I got the feeling their questions weren't being answered at all. They were being told the same thing over and over: "We can't answer that because we don't know." A lot of local people felt that the way they presented the information was immature, and that made people even more afraid. Yes, the situation is unknown, and no one knows what will happen, but they could have presented it in a more professional way, so it didn't scare people. Many local people felt they didn't have a PR person telling them what to say. If the government had presented the information in a better way, maybe we could have absorbed it and felt more comfortable.

'The scariest thing was not knowing which news source to trust, so after I while I stopped reading the news and following the numbers. Some media talked about medical information, but they weren't official medical centres. They'd say things that made me very worried and uncertain. I decided I'd better not read the news because I couldn't control it anyway.

'More and more people began getting the vaccine. I still needed to go to work and see people every day, and I worried that if I got COVID I'd pass it to my family and even my dog, because my dog is old and I'm very close to him. My parents were worried that if my dog caught COVID he might pass it to humans, so I bought a COVID test kit for my dog. I took a salvia sample from him and mailed it to the lab. I wanted to prove that the dog was clean.

'I delayed taking the vaccine until the last possible moment and finally got it in January 2022. I was very nervous. The only reason I got the second vaccine is that if I hadn't, I wouldn't have been able to go to restaurants or even the supermarket. I had a little dizziness after the second shot and sat in the vaccination facility for 45 minutes. I didn't faint, but when I got home, I was seeing in black and white. I sat on the floor; I didn't want to move. I didn't even dare to climb into my bed. That scared me and is the reason why I don't want to have the third vaccine. I got a medical exemption letter.'

***Ms Li** (not her real name), an event marketing manager in her 40s, relocated to China with her team in July 2020, when social distancing measures halted their projects in Hong Kong. She initially planned to stay two months but ended up spending more than two years in China, including several months in hotel quarantines. Despite being typically calm and rational, the extended periods of isolation and constant uncertainty took a toll on her mental health and eroded her resilience.*

'We went to Shanghai for an online movie project. There were a lot of procedures we needed to go through at the airport before we were directed to a place where we had to wait for a coach to take us to the quarantine hotel. Part of me was excited, and the other part was worried, because I didn't know what would happen next, or how long I'd be there. It was a totally unknown situation. In Hong Kong, when you did quarantine, you knew which hotel you would stay at because you booked it in advance, but in China it was a lottery. If you were lucky you got a five-star hotel, but if not, you were put in a hostel. I was expecting the worst but hoping for the best.

'I quarantined seven times over more than two years. The shortest was two weeks and the longest was 50 days. My first quarantine was for 14 days, and I got a three-star hotel which was clean. My worst quarantine was in Sanya, where I was given a dark and dirty room. I didn't want to sleep in the bed because there were bedbugs.

'The biggest problem for me was the constant uncertainty. If I knew I was going into a 21-day quarantine, then that was okay because I was mentally prepared. But what was really hard was when I was expecting quarantine to end and then got a call saying it would be extended another week, and then another week.

'In February 2022, I landed in Shanghai and needed to do a 21-day quarantine. By the time my quarantine finished, Shanghai had gone into lockdown. Everything was closed—all the shops, restaurants, and public transport. I was working online and by phone and email. The situation was constantly changing, and I couldn't predict what would happen the next day. It meant that I couldn't plan anything; I was just dealing with the situation from one day to the next. Not being able to grasp the whole situation made me really anxious and ungrounded. I felt so helpless; it was scary. I didn't know how to cope with the situation, but I still needed to be positive and deal with things as they came.

'My colleagues can normally control their emotions quite well, but during that time they lost their temper easily. I have quite a calm personality, but in this unpredictable situation I had my fears. My colleagues kept coming to me with questions, which increased my own fears. We needed to do a PCR test every day in the quarantine hotel. The nurse was supposed to come in the morning, but because there were so many people in the hotel they often didn't come at the scheduled time. When the nurse didn't come, my colleagues would panic and call me. I had no idea when the nurse would come, and when I couldn't give them an answer, I felt frustrated.

'The evening meal was supposed to come at 6 pm and when it didn't, everyone in the group would have a discussion on social media. There was a hotline to call, but it was always busy. I was facing lots of question, and I couldn't answer them, which made me feel hopeless. Everyone in the group knew they couldn't get an answer; they were just expressing themselves.

'The constant uncertainty became a mental challenge and I started questioning life. Why had I put myself in this situation? Why did this happen? The first two weeks in quarantine were okay, but after that I started to have strong emotions. I don't usually cry easily, but during that period I cried every morning. It became almost a routine. I cried, and then went back to face the wall. And the next day, I cried again. I couldn't tell my colleagues because I had a work image to maintain. The crying was something I could only share with myself, and later with a few close friends.

'I needed to communicate with my colleagues in Hong Kong. They didn't understand the situation we were facing, and that was a challenge. The common-sense view was that I was in a room by myself, so I must have plenty of time. They didn't understand that I was dealing with a lot of things. Just chasing the meal could take two to three hours a day. Something so simple could take so much time. Even if you got through to someone on the hotline and they said the meal was coming, that was two hours wasted. People who weren't in the same situation didn't understand. Luckily, I have a couple of friends who are good listeners, and I called them every day. Even though they had never experienced quarantine in China, they listened to my situation.

'In the first year of the pandemic, everyone thought the border with Hong Kong would reopen later that year. The next year, we expected it to open very soon. We waited almost three years for it to open. I didn't know when the situation would end, but I knew I had to get out of the situation. In the summer of 2022, I decided to quit. I came back to Hong Kong and now work for a charity. When the next pandemic comes, it would be good if people who are not going through unpredictable quarantines have a better understanding of what it is like. With more education and understanding, they might have more empathy.'

***Ma Jeuk** (not her real name) is in her late 20s and lives with her parents and husband in Chai Wan, at the eastern end of Hong Kong Island. She works for an organisation that supports farmers in the New Territories and is environmentally conscious.*

'I am very anti-vaccine. It's not that I don't want to cooperate with the government; it's because the vaccine is so new and there are so many uncertainties. It doesn't make sense to force people to do it. I felt quite angry because you have no choice. They tried so hard to force people to take the vaccine that it made me quite rebellious. In the beginning, it was quite easy to find a doctor to give you a certificate exempting you from taking the vaccine. It cost HK$500. Then the police clamped down on those doctors and many were no longer willing to do it, so the price went up to HK$3,000 for those who would still do it. That just shows that if you are rich enough you can survive.

'My husband is a teacher and because he chose not to get vaccinated, he had to do a PCR test every three days to go into school. My mum works in the healthcare system and was worried she'd lose her job if she couldn't get [an exemption] certificate. Even with the doctor's paper, she still needed to do a PCR test every week. Both my parents have heart problems. My dad is retired, and my mum was really anxious about getting infected at work and giving it to Dad. Her anxiety affected me. I wore a fabric mask—disposable paper masks create so much waste—and she was always on at me to wear a surgical mask.

'On Chinese news and social media, I often saw people sharing how to get masks and toilet paper. If you are into social media, this news pops up every day and you can't help but get affected and caught up in the storm. The darkest times were when everyone was so scared, the atmosphere was one of panic; people were going crazy in supermarkets and buying up all the toilet paper and stockpiling things at home. It created a lot of anxiety. I began thinking I should get some toilet paper. I knew I should act more rationally, but when the whole society is becoming irrational you start thinking you should follow. I had friends who stayed up all night searching the internet for how to buy masks from online Japanese stores. They spent HK$200 on one box. This was for middle class, wealthier families. It was crazy—you use up all the masks in your country and you try to take masks from other countries. On Facebook, there were online sellers saying they had some masks left for sale, and people were posting in the comments section to reserve boxes. I saw so many people making requests and got caught up in the storm and left a comment to reserve two boxes, but I never got a response. People were so irrational at this time; you couldn't help getting pulled into the storm.

'My whole family got infected in March 2022. Because we weren't vaccinated, we had to stay at home for two weeks. Four people in a 400-square-foot flat for two weeks was a bit crowded. We have family nearby who sent us food to cook, and we ate together and played board games, so it was fine for me. Then I had the proof that I'd had COVID and didn't need to get vaccinated for six months. Just when that proof was about to expire, I got COVID for a second time. I guess my immune system is quite weak. This time a friend let us isolate at her house, which has a small garden. My husband and I went there for two weeks. It was much better than the first time. We were in the countryside, the air was good, and we could get some sunshine in the little garden. It was like a staycation. We were lucky to stay there, but it made me think about the people who didn't have this opportunity. There is so much inequality and injustice in society, and the pandemic really magnified this.

'Life is so much better and easier for the rich; that makes me angry. I live in Chai Wan, which is not a wealthy area. Even three months after the lifting of the mask mandate, I see many people in my neighbourhood still wearing masks, but in Central many people take their masks off. I think it's about class. The grassroots people need to work, and if they get sick, they can't work. Also, compared to more wealthy people, the health of the grassroots people is not as good. I live close to friends and family, and we have a small support network, so whenever we got sick or the other friends or family got sick, we could help to buy things and send them food. This was really important, the sharing of resources. We didn't really share a lot, but knowing that you have friends who can help you in the hard times helps a lot psychologically.'

***Jo Jo** (not her real name) was born and raised in Hong Kong and works in the arts. Two months before the start of the pandemic, her daughter was born with a rare disease. For the first three years of the little girl's life, she and her husband were regulars at Queen Mary Hospital. The potentially fatal condition was frightening, but it was the uncertainty about the constantly changing hospital policies that Jo Jo found most stressful.*

'My daughter was born at the end of the social movement in November 2019. She has a long-term illness—biliary atresia—which affects the liver and meant she needed surgery two months after she was born. Parents are usually allowed to visit the children's ward

24/7, and there's no limit to the number of family members who can come during the twice-daily visiting hours, but it was the start of the pandemic, and the hospital policy changed. Only two carers were allowed to visit a child, and they could only visit one at a time for 12 hours. Fortunately, I work in the arts and have flexible hours. My husband and I took it in turns to be with her for 12-hour shifts. We barely got any sleep. Most of the kids in the ward had long-term illnesses, and many of their parents worked full-time and the kids were alone in the ward. Throughout the pandemic, there were a few episodes, which meant she had to go to the hospital for two weeks or more each time.

'After her initial surgery, there was a face mask shortage, and we desperately looked for supplies. Our friends knew about our situation and gave us a lot of protective stuff. I was really stressed about getting infected at the hospital because Queen Mary was taking COVID patients. If we got COVID, it would mean we wouldn't be able to accompany her, and we didn't want to infect her. Many people said hospital toilets were the place of highest risk for COVID, so I didn't go to the toilet during my 12-hour shift.

'We stayed at home for most of the first year, aside from hospital visits and the occasional stroll in an open area. When she was six months old, whenever we went for a check-up, we let her wear a mask. In the beginning, it was hard to buy face masks for a baby, and then we found them online from a Korean supplier. Gradually, smaller face masks came on the market in Hong Kong.

'When my girl had her first episode after the surgery, she was admitted to hospital as an emergency case. My husband and I weren't able to accompany her without a negative PCR test. This meant going to a community centre and waiting more than a day to get the result. We were really stressed about our daughter being alone in the hospital. She was only a year old and sick; being separated from her parents was very scary for her. It was also really scary for us because she was so unwell.

'When she was one and a half, she suddenly went very pale and almost passed out. We rushed her to hospital and waited more than half a day before she was admitted. She had an acute liver infection. My husband rushed to the community centre to do a PCR test so that one of us would be able to go on the ward with her. The hospital staff were professional, but they were very stressed. One-third to one-half of the team were transferred to a "dirty team", to treat COVID patients, and they were short-staffed. The ward we usually went to was being used as a COVID ward, so we were transferred to another floor where the nurses and doctors were adapting. They were pushing out less serious patients to ease the stress on the staff. The staff were supposed to be working in shifts, but we saw the same nurses all the time.

'The most stressful part of the whole experience was the uncertainty, because we were never sure of the hospital policy and whether it would change suddenly. The access to information was very difficult. We relied on asking a parents group—parents of children with the same disease—and posted questions and shared information. People posted questions such as "Do you need to be vaccinated for a check-up?" or "Do you need a negative test result for a check-up?". None of us were sure of the current hospital policy. When the hospital began accepting rapid tests to gain access to the building, it meant we didn't need to keep going to community centres and waiting for results, which saved us a lot of time.

'We had very strong family support. In March 2022, during the fifth wave, my husband and I got COVID. My parents lived in our flat in Sai Ying Pun with our daughter, and my husband and I stayed at their place. A few days later, our daughter got infected, and so did my mum. By then, I was negative, and returned to take care of my daughter. The symptoms were not very serious for us.

'My daughter is now three and a half and her liver indexes have been stable for the last six months. She started school in September and is doing well. At home she doesn't wear a mask, but when she leaves home, she insists on wearing one and only takes it off to eat and drink. When we are playing outdoors, I don't wear a mask and encourage her to take hers off, but she wants to wear it. To her it's part of her outfit, like wearing clothes. She insists, and I respect her choice. She has always worn a mask and is very sensitive to smells if she takes it off. The smell of the street, gasoline, restaurants—for her it is overwhelming. It's one of the main reasons she wants to wear a mask even though it is so hot.'

* * *

Uncertainty can increase stress, undermining resilience and making it harder to cope with daily life. It is not one swift blow but rather a slow wearing away. Two years into the pandemic, and no end in sight, many who had never experienced mental health issues found themselves struggling to cope. As humans, we crave certainty—our ability to predict future outcomes has helped us thrive. But when the future is uncertain, anxiety can take over, heightening our stress response and causing irritability and even violent behaviour.

Uncertainty can also be generated and exaggerated by the media. Stories on worst-case scenarios and half-truths and rumours circulating on social media easily trigger panic and draw others into the fear frenzy. A paper by specialists at the Hong Kong Children's Hospital found that Hong Kong media reports on death following vaccination had the detrimental effect of aggravating the public's vaccination hesitancy (Leung & Hon, 2021).

News stories and social media hype sparked several waves of panic buying during the pandemic. First, it was face masks, then toilet paper, rice, and water. People queued overnight for goods. There was even an armed robbery at a Mong Kok supermarket over toilet rolls (Woodhouse, 2020).

According to Hong Kong clinical psychologist Dr Cindy Chan, panic buying is about people trying to reclaim a sense of control (Whitehead, 2020). In a world turned upside down, it is a way to reassure ourselves that we are doing something to keep ourselves and our families safe. But while this protective behaviour may seem proactive and supportive on the surface, it can ultimately keep us locked in a cycle of anxiety. There were so many unsettling factors about the COVID-19 outbreak—the increasing death toll, people having to work from home, and schools being suspended—that people had the sense they were losing control of their life.

We all respond differently to stress and uncertainty, shaped by our upbringing, personality, and experiences. While we may not always be aware of our coping style, it's possible to change it if it's not helpful. The suggestions below offer a starting point for managing uncertainty and stress.

Strategies and Support

Uncertainty can leave us feeling depressed and hopeless about the future. It can magnify the scope of our problems and paralyse us from taking action. The pandemic presented a multitude of uncertainties, and many found themselves consumed by worry. It's easy to believe that by worrying, we're actively keeping danger at bay and working towards a solution. However, chronic worrying is unproductive when events are beyond our control. It can exacerbate anxiety, drain our energy, and even lead to insomnia.

In times of uncertainty, it's easy to feel overwhelmed by the things we can't control. The pandemic brought with it a host of things that are outside our control, from the spread of the virus to job loss and changing government policies. But even in the face of these challenges we are not powerless. The first step is to accept that there are things beyond our control. Then focus on what you can change.

We can take small steps to improve our physical and mental health, such as exercising regularly, eating well, and staying connected with loved ones. These actions can help us feel more in control and better equipped to handle uncertainty. If you've lost your job or your income has taken a hit, focus on updating your resume, reaching out to professional contacts, and searching for work online.

Looking after our mental health means acknowledging our emotions. During a pandemic when there are so many unknowns, it is natural to feel anger. But anger can often mask more vulnerable emotions such as fear, anxiety, shame, sadness, and frustration. It is important to recognise that anger is a valid emotion and to gently explore what other emotions may be hiding beneath it. Some people may try to hide the way they are really feeling, believing that appearing strong is the best way to cope. However, it's natural to feel anxious and overwhelmed in the face of uncertainty, and bottling it up for too long can lead to burnout.

Pay attention to your body's signals. Are your shoulders tight? Are you holding your breath? These are signs that you may be feeling anxious. Allowing yourself to experience your emotions, even if they are uncomfortable, can help reduce stress.

Rather than worrying about the future, try to focus on the present moment. Mindfulness is a practice that involves intentionally directing your attention to the here and now. By doing this regularly, you can prevent negative thoughts from spiralling out of control and reduce stress levels. This can help you approach the situation with a clear and calm mind.

A natural response to uncertainty is to gather information by following the news closely. However, constantly checking the news can lead to increased anxiety. Consider limiting your news consumption to once or twice a day, and make sure to get your information from reputable sources. During the pandemic, fake news stories circulating on social media added to the panic, so be mindful of what you share with your friends and family.

By focusing on what we can control and taking care of ourselves, we can build resilience and navigate uncertain times with greater confidence.

11

Suicide

As the rest of the world began to open up and travel resumed in 2022, Hong Kong faced its darkest hour of the pandemic. After two years of restrictions and widespread fear, the mood was sombre and people's nerves were frayed. It was in this climate of uncertainty that COVID-19 began to spread rapidly in the community. While deaths from the virus had been low, suddenly the numbers escalated. By mid-March, Hong Kong recorded the highest number of COVID-19 deaths per population size in the world, a rate of more than 25 deaths per 100,000 residents—even higher than when the Omicron variant first appeared in the UK in 2021 (Taylor, 2022).

In this climate of fear, exhaustion, and uncertainty, the city saw an increase in people taking their own lives. The charity Suicide Prevention Services received 22,000 calls to its hotline in the first two months of 2022, a 50 percent increase over the previous two years. Local media ran stories of suicide attempts, and the Hong Kong Jockey Club Centre for Suicide Research and Prevention at the University of Hong Kong sounded the alarm. Its Suicide Index had reached 'crisis level'. In the seven days from March 22, there were 21 news reports about people killing themselves. The centre's director, Professor Paul Yip Siu-fai, warned that if the trend continued the number of suicides would surpass the 1,264 deaths during the 2003 SARS crisis (Yau, 2022).

Forty-year-old ***Tai Lui*** *(not his real name) was living a modest, stable life working as a mechanic and living alone in Kowloon. However, when the pandemic struck, he lost his job and became homeless. Estranged from his family, his life quickly spiralled. He chose the pseudonym 'Tai Lui' because it means 'out of the depth of misfortune comes bliss'.*

'At the start of the pandemic, I was living on the top floor of a walk-up building in Prince Edward and working for the Cross Harbour Tunnel. My job was to retrieve the vehicles that broke down in the tunnel. I'd been in the job almost seven years and enjoyed it. A year into the pandemic, in 2021, two of my colleagues got COVID and died suddenly. I knew them and was really shocked and sad. They were only their early 30s and vaccinated. Both of them lived in a hotel on Tsing Yi Island. I don't know why they got COVID. My boss wanted me to move onto their team to replace one of them. I didn't want to. I was very sad and afraid, so I quit my job.

'I tried to pick up some work, mostly part-time construction jobs here and there. After I left the Cross Harbour Tunnel job, I couldn't afford my rent. I'm not in contact with my family; it's been that way for many years. I had nowhere to go and had the idea of living on the rooftop of the building where I'd been renting. I found some black canvas and made a shelter, a bit like a tent. I started living on the rooftop in July 2021 and stayed there for nine months. Living outside, under the sun and the rain, it was like camping. I took my showers at a local community sports centre. For quite some time no one seemed to notice, or care, that I was there.

'My time living on the rooftop was tough, but it wasn't the most difficult time in my life. I've been through worse. Then I lost my wallet with my ID card and driving licence. That really stressed me out. I needed to replace the cards. I knew if I didn't, it would be hard to get another job. I didn't have friends to turn to for help. In the pandemic, everyone had things going on and they were focused on their own problems. My stress got worse. I started thinking, "What if I was dead?" I spent four days just lying under the canvas, not getting up to eat or anything. I only sipped a little water. I didn't want to do anything; I was very down. I thought about ending my life—it would be very easy to do it quickly. But then I thought I should try everything to stay alive before doing anything like that.

'My thoughts were going around and around my head, and I couldn't sleep. I didn't know what was going on with me. I wondered if I had a mental problem, so I went to Yau Ma Tei Specialist Clinic. I spoke to the nurse and told her I'd been having negative thoughts and couldn't sleep at night. She said, "You look ok." That was it. I'd tried to get help, and they didn't think I needed the service. It made me feel even more helpless. It seemed there was nothing I could do.

'After more than six months living on the roof, someone noticed that I was staying there illegally. The landlord of the top flat was legally responsible for the rooftop. They sent him a letter, and I was evicted. I tried to claim social welfare allowance, but my previous salary was more than the amount allowing me to get the benefit. I was referred to ImpactHK, an NGO that helps the homeless, to assess my situation. ImpactHK let me stay in their hostel. In August 2022, I got a job working at ImpactHK, helping manage the activities at the sports centre. I would rather work than claim a government benefit.

'In December 2022, my roommate at the hostel got COVID, and I tested positive as well. I was sent to Penny's Bay. It was beautiful, not a bad experience at all. I was given three meals a day. I could order cup noodles or whatever I needed from an app, and they delivered it quite quickly. I just relaxed and watched movies.

'If I met someone in the same position I was in—someone who lost their job and was homeless—I'd tell them to talk to someone to share their problems and try to seek help. If you don't do that, there's no way out. At least if you share with someone, there's a chance that things might get better. If you don't share, then nothing will change. It's easy to say, "Just talk to someone." But if you've tried and are rejected, it feels easier not to. The case worker at ImpactHK was kind and really listened. That helped me open up and be more willing to share.'

***Matt** moved from Hong Kong to his native Ireland with his Chinese wife and their young daughter. However, his wife struggled to adjust to life in Ireland, and they returned to Hong Kong in late 2019. Matt had secured a position as a NET teacher (native-speaking English teacher), but when the pandemic hit the offer was withdrawn. Unemployed and living with his mother-in-law in a small flat in a remote New Territories village, his marriage crumbled, and he fell into depression.*

'I wasn't working and had a lot of negative feelings about myself. I was getting more and more depressed, acting out and getting emotional. My grandfather died, and my aunt died a week later. I couldn't go to the funerals in Ireland, so I watched them online. Seeing people being emotional but having the support of others made it worse because I felt so alone.

'I got a job in September [2020] as a NET teacher, but it was tough because we were doing online learning. Even when I went to work, I wasn't socialising with people. I felt more isolated. I was unhappy, and my wife was unhappy. We were drifting further and further apart, and she started a relationship with someone else.

'The worst part was in March [2021], when we broke up, and I had to move out and be on my own. I got a small place nearby to be close to my daughter, but it was in a remote part of Yuen Long, and my friends didn't want to travel all the way out there. I had a ton of financial pressure, plus the pressure of separation. Everyone in the village is local or they know my ex-wife; I felt cut off from everyone. I only saw my friend for one or two hours a week; it was very isolating.

'I was terrified of testing positive, especially if I'd been around my daughter. At the time, they were separating kids from parents. She was only six at the time, and I didn't want to send her alone into a hospital system where the staff were overworked and stressed. Seeing different rules for people who were rich or in government made me feel worse. It was stressful. It wasn't fair.

'My dad in Ireland tried to commit suicide, and my mum had her own emotional issues because of my dad's situation. Then my sister had a baby and broke up with her partner. There was all this going on back home, and I was stuck in Hong Kong by myself. My family couldn't come to visit me because of quarantine, and I couldn't go there. Although I could have afforded the flight, I couldn't afford the time or the cost of three weeks in hotel quarantine. I asked my doctor about mental health support. He said if I went through the public system, I'd be on the waiting list for months and advised me to go private. But private therapy costs about HK$2,000 an hour. Unless you are in a well-paying job, it's impossible to get the support you need.

'I was by myself for two years with all these things going on. It was so isolating and tough. I was worried about money and my daughter and whether she'd forget me if my ex got a new partner. It reached boiling point in October 2021, when my ex told me her boyfriend was going to move in. That broke me. I felt very alone. It was the lowest I've ever felt, and I tried to end my life. A friend noticed something I'd written on a group chat and thought it was off. He got to my place 10 minutes after I'd taken the pills. He helped me. I took the next day off work and told the other NET teacher at my school. The panel head at the school offered support through the church, but I'm not religious, so I didn't take it.

'My friend stayed at my place for two weeks and put me in touch with affordable counselling at St John's Counselling Service, which was a lifesaver. When the hotel quarantine was dropped, my mum came to see me. I went to the airport to meet her and hugged her and cried for 10 minutes. She was here for six weeks with my daughter and me, which was amazing.

'I still have days when I feel awful and depressed, but I'm in a better place now and am in a new relationship. Things improved with counselling and as the COVID restrictions started to wind down. Looking back, I would have liked to have seen some leeway in the restrictions for people who had big things going on in their life, like divorce or a family member passing away. A system where people could apply for home quarantine, or a travel subsidy, or get help getting back on track, would have been really good. More affordable mental health support is needed in Hong Kong.'

***Kim-fai** (not her real name) was 61 years old in 2019, when the legal firm she worked for relocated to Singapore, prompting her to retire. She lived in Sha Tin with a full-time domestic helper and was active in her church. However, when the pandemic hit, she was isolated at home. A series of setbacks led her to a dark place, and she attempted suicide.*

'The protests in 2019 were really frightening. There were young people running in the streets; everything was so destructive. My legal firm relocated to Singapore, but I didn't want to leave. I was born in Hong Kong; it's the only home I've ever known. I'm too old to move to a new place, so I was forced to retire. My husband and I have been separated for 20 years. He has a live-in girlfriend, but we didn't divorce. Sometimes I needed financial support, but my husband ignored me and broke off the communication. My daughter is now in her 30s. She suffered because she got caught in the middle between my husband and me.

'After I retired, I lived in a flat in Sha Tin with my maid, and my daughter would come to see me. Then the pandemic started, and I felt really miserable. Hardly anyone went out; they just ran to the shops to get the daily necessities and hurried home. People were very scared. I was in a very lonesome place and was hiding by myself. The maid who had been working for me for over 20 years retired because her son was getting married. My relationship with my daughter deteriorated, and we were critical of each other. Everything was so negative. Because of my family problems, and everything that was happening in the city, I stayed home alone.

'I used to be very involved with the church, but with COVID I was completely solitary. It was a very difficult time, and I was just counting my fingers day and night. In February 2022, during the fifth wave, things were very bad. A lot of the elderly people I knew through the church died. I kept hearing about this auntie dying and that uncle passing away. I began thinking that life was meaningless. Every night when I tried to sleep, I couldn't stop crying. My pillow was wet with tears.

'One day, I became out of control, and fell from a height of 20 metres. It was a miracle I survived. I was taken to the Prince of Wales

Hospital. My pelvis was broken, both the left and right sides, and both my ankles were smashed. It was only when I was moved out of intensive care, five days after my fall, that I realised how serious my situation was. The consultant said if I'd fallen on my head instead of my feet I would have died instantly.

'I had eight surgeries, and they put titanium screws in my hips and ankles. The medical team were amazing. The psychiatrist diagnosed me as still under SP [suicidal possession]. I told him my fears and worries—suicide is considered a sin by the church. After talking to him for some days, I told him I wanted religious support. A father from the church came to visit me. Speaking to the father helped to erase some of my worries. I was hospitalised for 140 days and then went to the rehabilitation hospital. I was in pain 24 hours a day. In the beginning I couldn't sleep more than one or two hours, but now I sleep better. I'm on a lot of medication for the pain; it's chronic.

'My brother brought me to stay in an elderly care home. He suggested that I try it for three months and see how I like it. It's been six months, and I feel like a family member. I would like to stay here. Some of the people in the care home are really quite sick, so in the morning I go around and talk to them. Some of them are blind, but now they recognise my voice. Small acts of kindness make them happy. I have a fantastic brother who helped me through all this. He visits me and brings me fruit salad and yoghurt. He is helping me work on my divorce. I should have got divorced a long time ago, and then I could have got remarried.

'I see a psychiatrist every two months. I'm now back to myself, and the depression is almost gone, but I still need to take sleeping pills. My daughter has PTSD. My brother suggested that I leave my daughter alone. She has all my blessings. I have forgiven myself, and I've done all the repentance to God to forgive me my sins. Now I'm a reborn child; I really want to achieve a lot. One day, when I don't need to rely on the wheelchair too much, I want to console people at funerals through the church. I want to tell them that life is meaningful. I want to visit elderly homes, and talk to the old people, and show a good heart and love. I want to play games with them and show them there is warmth in the world.'

* * *

The pandemic had a significant impact on the elderly, particularly men. The constant fear of contracting the virus, coupled with the isolation and loneliness brought on by social distancing measures, led to an increase in elderly people taking their lives. The suicide rate of men aged 60 and above jumped from 24.3 per 100,000 people in 2020 to 27.3 in 2021. Meanwhile, the suicide rate of elderly women saw a slight decrease from 14.9 in 2020 to 14.6 in 2021 (University of Hong Kong, 2022a).

Depression is one of the most common mental health issues among elderly people; typically one in 10 older adults is affected. But that figure increased during the pandemic. In the immediate wake of the fifth wave, a study of almost 5,000 elderly people found that one-third were suffering from anxiety, depression, or loneliness—or a combination. Their biggest concern, they said, was that they would be a burden on their families if they were infected with COVID-19 (University of Hong Kong, 2022b).

There was also an alarming increase in suicides among children under the age of 15, boys being particularly at risk. The suicide rate of boys doubled from 1.2 in 2020 to 2.4 in 2021, reaching an historic high. The rate for girls decreased slightly from 1.2 in 2020 to 1.0 in 2021. Girls and young women aged 15 to 24 experienced a sharp increase in suicide rates, the rate rising from 4.4 in 2019 to 6.0 in 2020, then to 6.5 in 2021.

The pandemic's severe disruption to schooling was a key trigger for the rise in students taking their own lives. The sudden switch to online classes and postponed exams left many struggling to adapt. The Hong Kong Jockey Club Centre for Suicide Research and Prevention analysed 36 student suicides between January 2021 and June 2022 and found that more than a quarter of the suicide notes mentioned academic stress.

The crushing weight of the pandemic was felt most acutely in working-class neighbourhoods, where small flats made social distancing difficult and tensions ran high. A 2022 study of 3,340 young people aged 15 to 24 found that 20 percent had contemplated suicide in the last year, 5 percent had made a plan to take their own lives, and 1.5 percent had attempted suicide (Hung, 2023). Those with major depressive disorder—the symptoms of depression last for at least two weeks and interfere with daily activities—were found to be three times more likely to have suicidal thoughts and eight times more likely to make a plan or attempt suicide. The highest rates of depression were seen in women aged 22 to 24 who also lived in public housing flats.

As the demand for mental health support surged, the public healthcare system struggled to keep up. Some people waited two years to get an initial consultation at a clinic, by which time many had lost the motivation to seek help. The majority of those with mental health issues haven't been able to get proper support. This problem doesn't just disappear; it festers, as seen in the alarming incidents of violence since COVID-19 restrictions were lifted.

Strategies and Support

The fear and social stigma concerning suicide often prevents us from addressing the issue head-on. We may shy away from discussing it with someone who could be at risk. But if we had a better understanding of how to identify those in danger and how to approach the conversation, we could save lives.

Changes in attitude or behaviour can be a warning sign. A person may sleep more or less than usual, become less concerned about their appearance, or may speak especially slowly or especially fast. They may experience depression, mood swings, or lose interest in social activities. They experience feelings of hopelessness and being a burden to others.

Certain individuals may be at higher risk. Those who are socially isolated, have strained family relationships, or have experienced abuse or bullying may be more vulnerable. Financial difficulties, substance abuse problems, and past suicide attempts can increase risk.

You don't need special training to offer someone emotional support; just listen non-judgementally. Although it can be upsetting to hear that someone you care about is distressed, try to stay calm. You are not trying to talk them out of the problem or solve it but being a container for their feelings.

Don't ask if they are okay—that will likely illicit a standard response. A simple, 'I've noticed you haven't been yourself recently; would you like to talk about it?' can open the door to a more meaningful conversation. Give them the time they need to respond, and remember not to blame or judge them for their feelings. It may have taken a lot of courage for them to open up to you.

It is a common misconception that asking someone directly about suicidal thoughts can plant an idea in their head. In reality, asking direct questions such as 'Are you having thoughts of ending your life?' can provide an opportunity for them to open up about their feelings. If they're not experiencing suicidal thoughts, they'll tell you right away. If they are, it's a chance to discuss getting professional help and support.

Some people believe that talking about suicide is just a cry for attention, but it's important to always take it seriously. It takes a lot of courage for someone to open up about their thoughts of suicide. If someone shares their thoughts with you, don't dismiss them or tell cheer up.

There is a common misconception that if someone feels suicidal then they will always feel that way. However, this is not true. With the right support it's possible to overcome these feelings. Suicide is preventable. If you are struggling with suicidal thoughts, it is important to reach out for help and share your feelings. It's ok to seek support, especially when things are overwhelming. If you don't feel comfortable speaking to a family member or a close friend, there are dedicated suicide hotlines staffed by trained volunteers who can provide support to people in crisis.

The Samaritans 24-hour telephone hotline / +852 2896 0000
The Samaritan Befrienders Hong Kong / +852 2839 2222
Suicide Prevention Services (24-hour) / +852 2382 0000

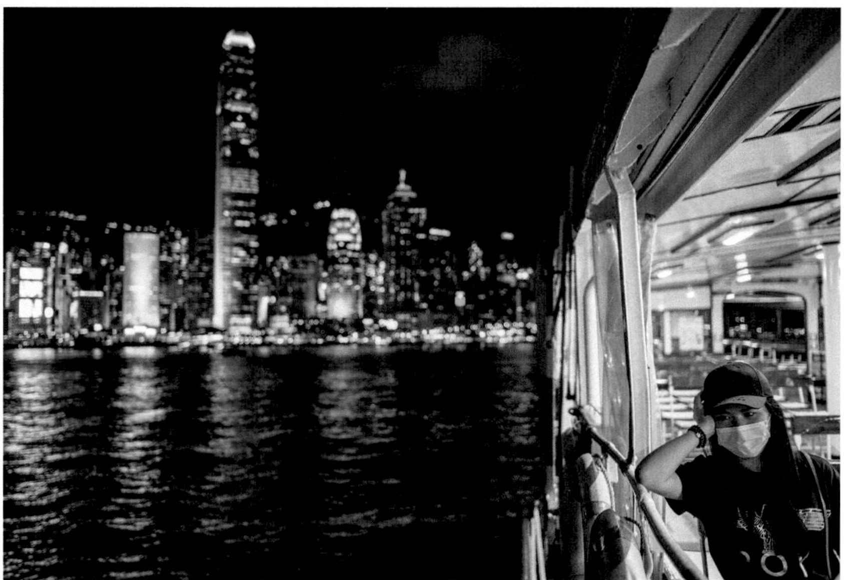

A woman crossed Victoria Harbour from Kowloon side to Hong Kong Island on the Star Ferry on July 27, 2020. It was the week that tough new social distancing measures were introduced and the wearing of masks in public was made mandatory. Photo by Anthony Wallace © AFP.

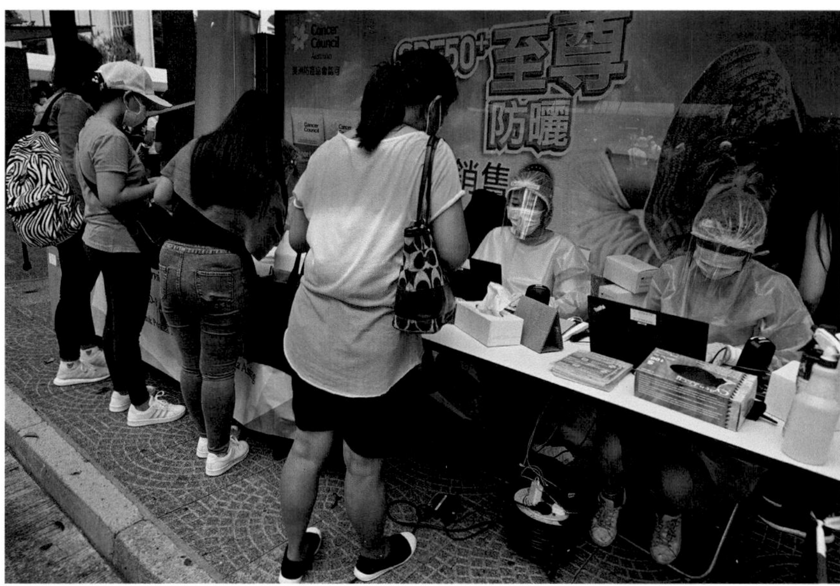

Migrant workers registered for COVID-19 testing in Central on May 1, 2021, after the government ordered all foreign domestic workers to get tested after two domestic workers who entered the city from overseas were found to be infected with a more infectious coronavirus variant. Photo by Peter Parks © AFP.

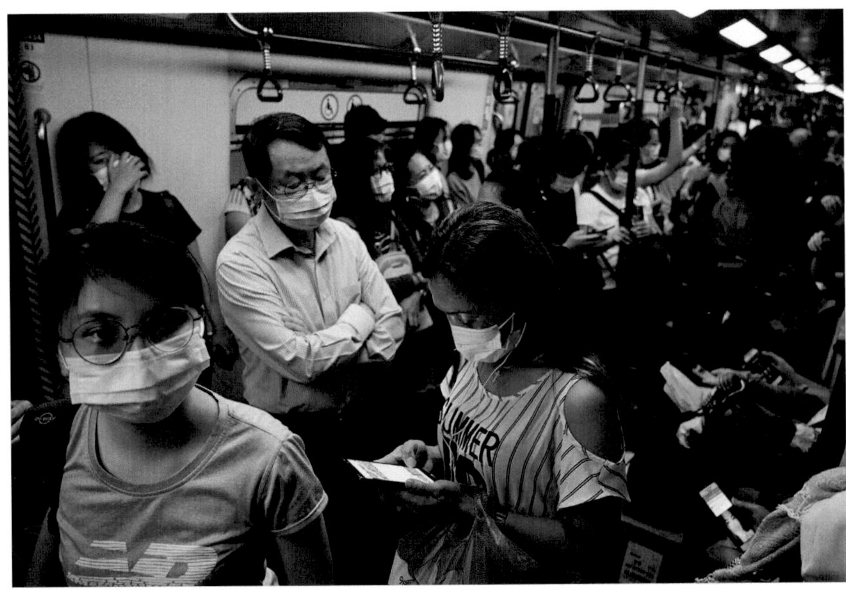

Masked commuters travelled by MTR on November 22, 2020 as a spike in COVID-19 cases brought in tighter restrictions and forced a planned travel bubble between Hong Kong and Singapore to be scrapped a day before its launch on November 21. Photo by Peter Parks © AFP.

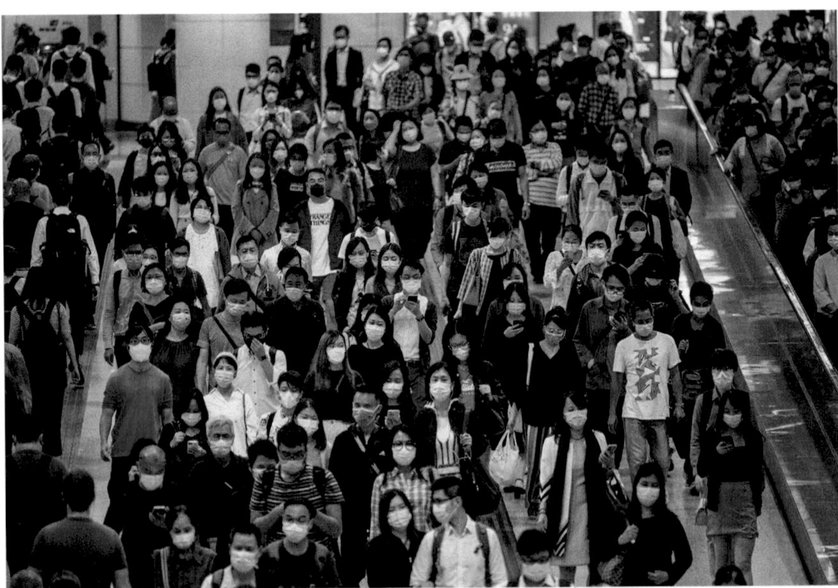

The mandatory wearing of face masks in public took effect in July 2020. When it was lifted almost three years later on March 1, 2023, many people continued to wear face masks in public. Photo by Anthony Wallace © AFP.

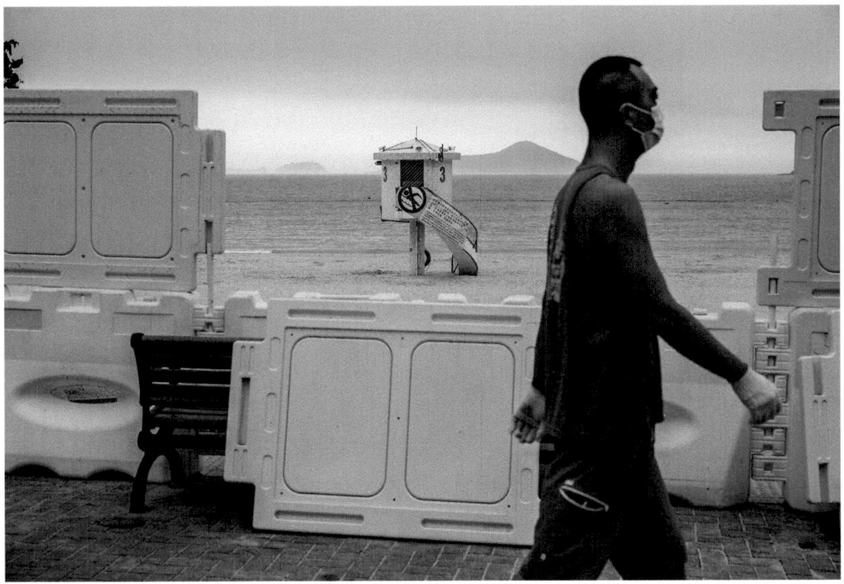

A worker put up a fence to block access to Shek O beach in Hong Kong on March 17, 2022 after the government said it would close public beaches to curb the spread of the virus. Photo by Dale de la Rey © AFP.

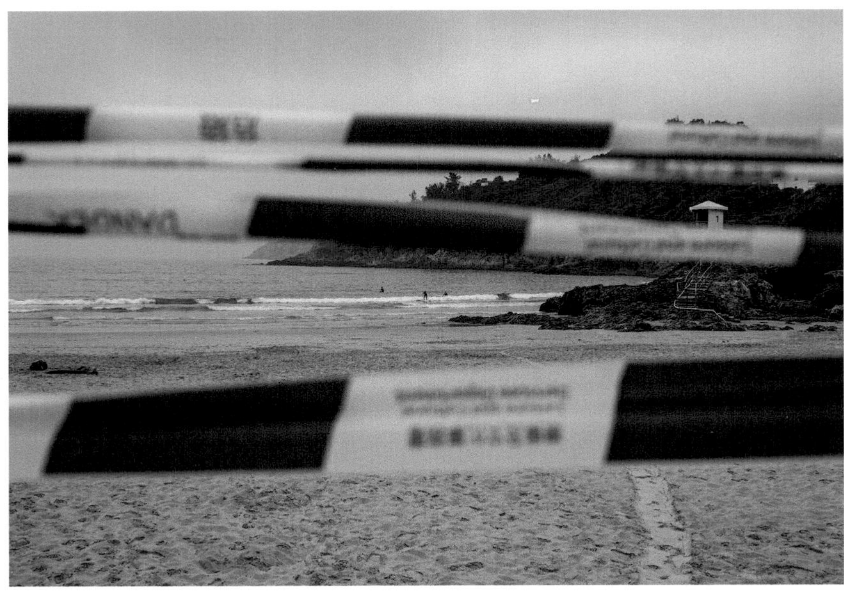

People surfed as workers started to close Big Wave Bay beach on March 17, 2022. All gazetted bathing beaches and outdoor leisure facilities were initially closed in December 2020 and reopened in April 2021 before being closed again in 2022. Photo by Dale de la Rey © AFP.

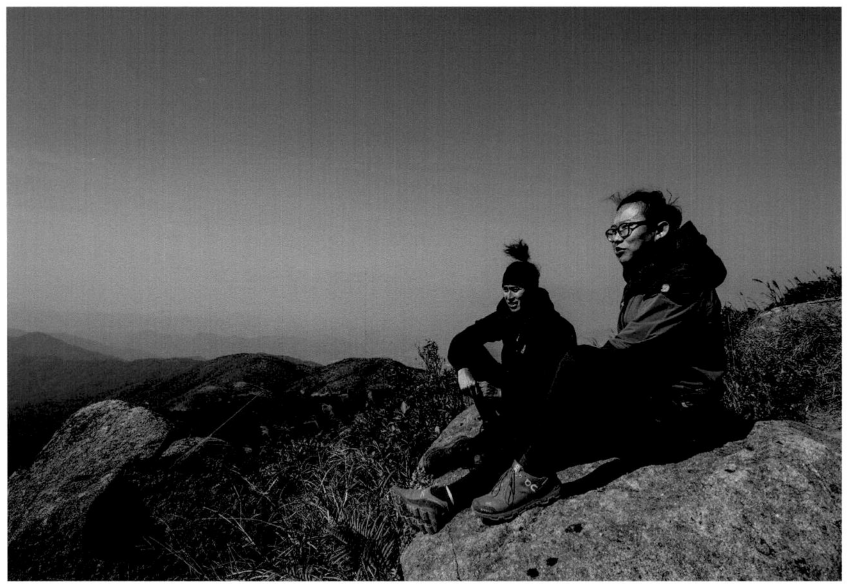

With sports facilities and the beaches closed, Hong Kong's trails became a popular destination for outdoor activities. At their most stringent, the restrictions required hikers to be accompanied by no more than one person. Photo by Anthony Wallace © AFP.

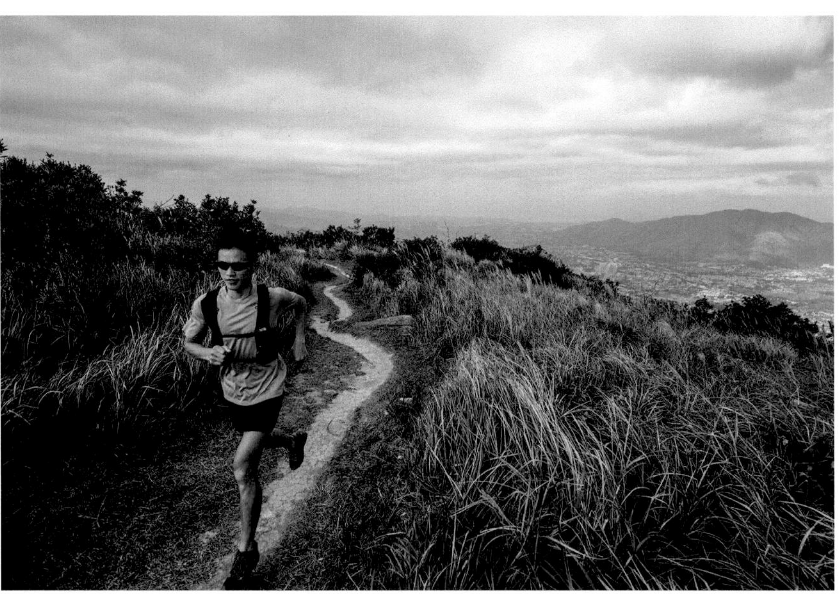

The pandemic brought a surge of hikers to Hong Kong's trails. In addition to the mental health benefits of being in a natural environment, the physical exertion of hiking also boosts psychological wellbeing. Photo by Anthony Wallace © AFP.

12

Nature as Healer

Hong Kong's lockdown experience was different from that of many other parts of the world. While residents in other countries were confined to their homes and only allowed brief excursions outside, those in Hong Kong were free to move about the city and visit the countryside albeit with restrictions in place. With sports facilities and the beaches closed, the trails became a popular destination for outdoor activities. At their most stringent, the restrictions required hikers to be accompanied by no more than one person and to wear a face mask at all times.

There's a significant link between mental health and engagement with our natural world. A study published in *Science Advances* found that spending time in natural environments can have a profound positive impact on our mental well-being. From reducing stress to boosting positive emotions, the possible psychological benefits of interacting with nature are numerous (Bratman et al., 2019).

Susannah Whyte *(not her real name), a 43-year-old marketing professional, found herself struggling with anxiety and panic attacks during* *the pandemic. But she discovered an unexpected source of strength and comfort: the great outdoors. Hiking became a regular part of her routine, and she credits the time spent in nature with providing her with a protective shield against the stresses of the world.*

'I started suffering from anxiety during the pandemic, which is something I'd not had before. When Hong Kong brought out the first quarantine, which was a home quarantine, we thought it would be temporary. My nan in the UK wasn't well. I was waiting for the home quarantine to finish so I could go and see her. When it didn't, I was very disappointed and had an emotional crash. After that, my approach was to assume the worst, because I didn't want to suffer from so many emotional rollercoasters. Hong Kong's rules kept changing and there were so many rumours. Constantly monitoring the situation and checking the news feeds was exhausting.

'I ended up doing a couple of hotel quarantines during the pandemic which affected my mental health. The first was a three-week quarantine and I prepared well. Friends dropped off food for me, I worked during the day and I exercised, but by day 14 it started getting hard. On day 17, the shower didn't work, and I had a complete meltdown. I managed to pick myself up. After that I spent a lot of time staring out the window. I was excited to leave quarantine, but the adjustment was hard. I felt as though I was learning to interact with people again.

'Seven months later, I did a one-week hotel quarantine. I thought it would be easy as it was just seven days, so I didn't prepare as I did for the first. When the quarantine hotel door slammed shut on me, my body went into shock. I think it was the after-effects of the first quarantine. I had PTSD. I found it really hard to get myself motivated, and one week in there felt like three weeks.

'I got my first panic attack during the pandemic. It came out of the blue, and it was only afterwards that I realised I'd had a panic attack. It happened when I was working from home. I began to feel really short of breath and panicky and had to lie on the floor. When the panicky feeling passed, I felt completely exhausted. It was the first of many panic attacks.

'It was about this time that I began having really bad period pains that left me doubled over for a couple of days. I went to see the doctor and all the tests came back negative. She asked me more about the symptoms, and I told her about the panic attacks and being teary and upset. She said she thought I was an emotionally strong person and the anxiety was manifesting in physical symptoms. She wanted to put me on medication, but I didn't want to take pills. I don't even like taking paracetamol. So, I went to see a counsellor. It was the best thing I've ever done.

'Within a few sessions with the counsellor, I learned some coping strategies. By identifying and naming what I was feeling, I was able to stop it tipping over into a full-blown panic attack. I learned to spot the signs much earlier and no longer got the awful feeling that I was falling off a cliff. I also started meditating and learned TRE (tension releasing exercises).

'The counsellor suggested that I identify things that make me happy. I told her I'd gone on a hike and really enjoyed it, and she encouraged me to hike more often. Being in nature is always wonderful. I feel that it tops up my energy levels and boosts my resistance. During the pandemic, hiking was a chance to get away from everything—the mask wearing, the rules, the police. It took me away from all the restrictions for a few hours, and I could talk to my friends about what was going on in my life, the world, and remember what an amazing place I live in.

'On a trail you bump into fellow hikers and give each other a smile or encourage each other up a hill; it felt good. Hiking became a regular thing during COVID. I would do one local hike on Lamma Island where I live and another longer hike elsewhere at the weekend with friends. I had a couple of groups of friends who regularly organised hikes, which helped push me to get out. Some days I might think I just want to rest at home on the sofa, but when I was out on a trail with friends, I felt much better. I'd carry that memory of the weekend hike through the week. Hiking became a necessary thing to do, and if I didn't do it, I could feel it.

'Sometimes I'd go for a swim in the sea as a way of throwing off the COVID stuff. We are surrounded by water, and getting access to the water is easy whether through the beach or water sports. It's hard to go anywhere in Hong Kong where you can't see the water or the hills. I was lucky to be living in a place where access to nature is easy. I totally credit it with helping me get through COVID and the panic attacks. Sometimes, if I felt uneasy, going for a walk or just looking out the window at nature could be enough to right my emotions. Being in nature gave me a forcefield of protection to bat away the negative things.'

***Heinok** was a recent graduate of Hong Kong University's dentistry programme and had just started her first job in dentistry when the pandemic struck. Her parents were living in Australia, and her brother was studying in the UK. She is a Mind HK ambassador.*

'Growing up, I was a perfectionist. I want everything to be done to the dot. When I've done something well, I scrutinise every little mistake rather than celebrate what I've done well. I'm the sort of person who gets nervous, especially when I don't know what will come next. The pandemic aggravated all that because there was so much uncertainty and time to think. I began ruminating about things in the past—personally and professionally.

'Very early on in the pandemic, they closed the dental clinics, which meant I wasn't able to work, and that led to financial stress. I worried about how I was going to afford my rent. My parents are in their 60s and living in Australia. My younger brother was studying in the UK and alone over there. We were worried about how to get him out. The rules and regulations were changing all the time. Not knowing what would happen made me very anxious. The day my brother was due to fly to Australia, they closed the border. My parents decided to stay in Australia. I was worried about them, especially my dad, who has underlying health conditions. If they needed help, they'd only have each other.

'I started a master's programme. It was a pretty intense course; the people on the programme are workaholics. My parents moved back to Hong Kong and got an apartment near where I was doing my masters. I moved in with them. When the guy who encouraged me to join the programme left Hong Kong, I began to really feel the pressure. I wasn't eating or sleeping well and was feeling the pressure of the school and courses. I got to a point where I was on a diet of coffee and bananas, so I decided to take a break and leave the programme. I fell into depression. I wasn't sure if I wanted to go back into dentistry. I began working at Lululemon and teaching yoga on the side. At the height of the pandemic, during the fifth wave, my mum was worried about me catching COVID and bringing it back to Dad. I was so stressed at the thought of giving him COVID that I moved out.

'I have a tendency that when I don't like things, I go away. But I couldn't do that during the pandemic because I was stuck in Hong Kong. The flats here are quite small, and if you're working from home or stuck at home in a small space it can have an impact on your mental health and make you feel claustrophobic. When I was growing up, we'd often hike outdoors as a family. When I'm outside, in nature, it helps ground me and makes me realise I'm part of a big world.

'What really saved me during the pandemic was hiking. My boyfriend is a fan of [Stanford University neuroscientist] Andrew Huberman and follows his well-being philosophy. He likes to hike on Sundays to set up his energy for the week. I usually hike with him or family and sometimes by myself. Outdoors the air is fresher, and it helps me with my nasal blockage. When I'm in the dental clinic, the sounds of people and equipment can be noisy. Being outdoors it's peaceful and allows me the space to think more quietly. When I'm in nature, surrounded by green, I start to relax. I find the quiet and the space that you get being in nature therapeutic.

'I avoid trails where there are a lot of people. I like to hike High West on the Peak and Lantau Peak. I also like the beginning of the MacLehose Trail, which has incredible views and you end up on the beach. I enjoy going up steps. It's good exercise and I like the reward at the top. Perhaps it's the high achiever in me; I like to see a nice view at the summit as I drink my water. We can sit a lot, so it's nice to move and release the tension in your shoulders and hips. When the restaurants and gyms were closed during the pandemic, more people began hitting the trails, and that has continued. I've noticed there are a lot more ribbon trails now than before the pandemic.'

* * *

Hong Kong is often associated with a bustling metropolis teeming with towering skyscrapers and throngs of people. However, this is only part of the city's true identity. In reality, Hong Kong's 7.4 million inhabitants occupy a mere 25 percent of its 1,108 square kilometres. The remaining expanse is a verdant oasis comprising country parks and protected areas. This juxtaposition means that urban dwellers are never more than a stone's throw from nature; within 30 minutes, one can trade the concrete jungle for a serene hiking trail.

S. K. Shum, a passionate hiker, has always believed in the power of open spaces to soothe the mind. During the SARS outbreak in 2003, he observed an increase in the number of hikers in Hong Kong and subsequently founded the Hong Kong Hiking Meetup group in 2005. Despite the fact that organised hikes were not possible during the pandemic, he once again witnessed a surge in interest in hiking. The group he founded describes itself as 'probably the largest hiking group in the world', and now has 27,000 members and organises 1,800 hikes per year.

In the 1970s, scientists began studying what Shum had intuitively sensed—that time spent in nature has a positive impact on our well-being. Their research showed that scenes of nature were associated with positive feelings of friendliness, affection, and joy (Summers & Vivian, 2018).

In 1982, the Japanese Forestry Agency coined the term *shinrin-yoku*—which is often translated as 'forest bathing'—in a dual campaign to encourage people to visit forests for their health and as a means of protecting the forests. *Shinrin-yoku* is the practice of mindfully immersing yourself in the atmosphere of the forest using all five senses. Studies on physical and mental health benefits report reduced stress, anxiety, and depression symptoms as well as improved mood and relaxation (Hansen et al., 2017).

In the early 1990s, the ecopsychology movement emerged with the goal of understanding and harmonising the relationship between humans and the earth. This movement suggests that disconnection from our natural surroundings can contribute to various mental health conditions. From this movement, ecotherapy was developed, which seeks to improve psychological functioning through the use of green spaces. The fundamental idea is that by immersing ourselves in nature, we become more connected and aware of our surroundings, leading us to question our existence beyond ourselves.

In 2019, a study was conducted to determine the optimal duration of time spent in nature for stress reduction. The study used cortisol, a hormone that indicates stress levels in the body, as a key indicator. The results showed that spending 20 to 30 minutes in nature significantly and efficiently reduced stress levels, an 18.5 percent drop in cortisol per hour. While the benefits continued to accrue after 30 minutes, the rate of cortisol reduction decreased to 11.4 percent per hour (Hunter et al., 2019).

In addition to the mental health benefits of being in a natural environment, the physical exertion of hiking Hong Kong's trails boosts psychological well-being. Aerobic exercises, such as walking and jogging, have been shown to reduce anxiety and depression. Exercise improves mood by enhancing self-esteem and cognitive function and can alleviate symptoms like low self-esteem and social withdrawal (Mikkelsen et al., 2017). Additionally, exercise promotes better sleep, which is crucial for reducing stress, anxiety, and depression. Exposure to sunlight is also beneficial, as it is thought to increase the brain's release of serotonin, a hormone associated with improved mood and feelings of calmness and focus.

Ecotherapy can also be practised indoors by observing nature through a window or bringing elements of nature, such as plants, inside. Environmental psychologists Rachel and Stephen Kaplan have attributed nature's restorative ability to something they termed 'soft fascination'. This concept suggests that observing natural phenomena, such as leaves rustling in the wind, or birds soaring through the sky, can replenish our capacity for attention and promote a sense of well-being. They argue that this type of engagement with nature can 'lull us into a sort of hypnotic state, where negative thoughts and emotions are overtaken by a positive sense of well-being' (Abrams, 2013).

During the pandemic, people who underwent the mandatory hotel quarantine quickly discovered the benefit of having a room with a view. Gazing out at the sea or a verdant landscape became a coveted luxury and hotels charged a premium for such rooms. Isolated for weeks on end, many longed for some connection to the living world. In an effort to ease their guests' confinement, two high-end quarantine hotels, the Ovolo and the Dorsett Wanchai, gifted them with potted plants. The benefits of this indirect contact nature were confirmed by researchers at Hong Kong University, who found that having a view of nature, whether it be the sea or a green mountainside, helped to mitigate the negative effects of the quarantine and reduce stress levels (Hazan & Chan, 2022).

The allure of nature's untamed beauty is undeniable. Its remote, wild, and unpredictable character can restore our psychological well-being. However, we can't go into it blindly. The very things that make nature so appealing can also be dangerous, especially for city dwellers unaccustomed to the great outdoors. The pandemic brought a surge of hikers to the trails, but with it came an increase in casualties. In 2022, requests for mountain search and rescue services rose to 600, up from 328 in 2020. Tragically, 12 people lost their lives in 2022, compared to 2 in 2020. And the number of injuries skyrocketed from 125 in 2020 to a staggering 325 in 2022 (Zhao, 2023).

Strategies and Support

There are countless ways to enjoy the benefits of being in nature. Whether it's scaling a mountain or simply basking in the sun, there is no one right way to experience the outdoors. The key is to find what brings you joy and happiness. If the thought of huffing and puffing up a steep hill fills you with dread, fear not. There are many other ways to commune with the natural world. Let your mood, the weather, and the season be your guide as you explore the many ways to interact with the natural world.

Engage in outdoor activities / Take a leisurely stroll through a country park or, for the more energetic, lace up your running shoes and hit the trails. Alternatively, a barefoot walk along the beach, feeling the sand between your toes, can create a feeling of being grounded while listening to the lapping of the waves can help reduce stress and anxiety. If you want to share the experience with others, gather some friends and enjoy a meal outdoors—there are plenty of designated barbecue and picnic spots in the parks and beaches. If you'd rather have some alone time, bring along a sketchbook and capture the beauty of nature with pencil and paper. The process of drawing and focusing on a particular scene can help calm a wandering mind.

Bring nature indoors / Visit the Mong Kok Flower Market, located just off Prince Edward Road. This market offers a wide selection of fresh flowers and potted plants at affordable prices. Studies have shown that being around flowers can reduce stress, enhance concentration, and improve mood. You can also incorporate nature into your workplace. Keeping a small potted plant on your desk and taking a few minutes to gaze at it can help reduce stress. And if you're on the go, you can also carry a slice of nature with you wherever you go by taking photographs of places and views that you enjoy and setting them as the background on your mobile phone. There are also many free apps available that offer a range of nature sounds, from the rustling of trees to waves lapping on the shore and thunderstorms. Choose a sound that you find soothing and play it when you are feeling anxious or having trouble falling asleep. Research has found that listening to recordings of nature can boost mood, decrease stress, and even lessen pain. Another simple way to connect with nature is by looking out the window and watching the clouds drift across the sky.

Help the environment / Joining a community litter pickup is a great way to help the environment and improve your mental health. Organisations such as Hong Kong Clean Up (http://hkcleanup.org), Plastic Free Seas (www.plasticfreeseas.org), and EcoMarine (www.ecomarinehongkong.org) organise regular events. Searching for litter requires concentration, which can distract you from worrisome thoughts and help you be in the present moment. You'll also meet new people and enhance your sense of belonging. Another way to support the environment is by volunteering with The Nature Conservancy (https://www.tnc.org.hk), which works to restore oyster reefs in Hong Kong. You can collect discarded oyster shells or remove invasive cordgrass that turns wet mudflats into dry land. Alternatively, you can volunteer at Kadoorie Farm and Botanic Garden (www.kfbg.org) by helping with their weekly farmers' market or assisting with planting and gardening work.

13

Silver Linings

The COVID-19 pandemic forced people to adapt quickly to unprecedented challenges: working from home, online schooling, tighter budgets, and job losses. While this book paints a grim picture of these challenges, it's important to also recognise the silver linings that emerged during this crisis. This chapter is not simply an attempt to lighten the mood, but rather an exploration of the importance of actively seeking out silver linings in even the darkest of times—a practice that can have profound benefits for our mental health.

It is important to note that experiencing moments of joy or positivity in the midst of hardship does not negate or erase the pain and suffering that may also be present. Positive and negative emotions can coexist, and finding moments of happiness does not mean ignoring or denying feelings of fear or grief.

During the SARS epidemic in 2003, some people experienced unexpected positive impacts on their mental health. According to a study by Lau et al. (2006), individuals felt more supported by their loved ones, paid closer attention to their own mental well-being, and even adopted healthier lifestyles. Similarly, another study found that SARS patients reported greater social connectedness, personal growth, and interpersonal appreciation as a result of their illness (Cheng et al., 2006). These positive changes emerged as individuals struggled to make sense of and find meaning in the distressing situation.

When the pandemic first hit in 2020, ***Jacqueline****, an educational psychologist, had a two-year-old son enrolled in a private nursery school. A year later, she gave birth to her daughter. But when her daughter was just six months old, the entire family was sent to a government-run quarantine camp. Despite the challenges, Jacqueline sees unexpected upsides to the experience—some of which have had long-lasting effects.*

'I feel the pandemic offered me more good things than bad. My son's nursery school set up Zoom classes. The lessons were done in a group of no more than eight students, and the teachers were caring and able to cater to their needs. I enjoyed working from home and being with my son, even doing the online classes with him. When I look back at those moments, I see they were really precious. There were lots of limitations and, of course, the social aspect could not be replaced, but it was brilliant as a parent to sit beside him and help him understand a little more. The school sent us a resource package every week with educational games to do with our kids to improve their fine-motor skills and help them recognise colours and shapes and learn new words. My son was young, and I enjoyed it. If I had been at work, I wouldn't have had that time with him; it was precious. I feel guilty when I consider that my daughter is now that age and I can't give her the same individual attention because I'm back in the office.

'During the pandemic, I worked from home more often and had more time to rest. My daughter, Jasmine, was born in June 2021. I wasn't stressed; I'd already had the experience of giving birth at the Queen Mary Hospital and went back there. Some of my friends who had their first child during the pandemic were really panicky because their husbands weren't allowed in the delivery room. I would have found that very stressful because I needed my husband's support. Fortunately, when Jasmine was born the restrictions weren't as stringent, and my husband was able to join me as long as he showed a negative COVID test.

'After a time, we switched our son to a government kindergarten. We wanted him to have more play-based sessions than the nursery school was able to offer, and we wanted him to be in a Christian school and learn more about the scriptures and God's love. I was shocked that they placed 30 kids in one online class. The school used Teams as its online platform, and the teacher and students were tiny squares on the screen. They couldn't see their classmates' faces clearly. We were sent resource packages, but not as many or as good as the ones the nursery school had provided. They did their best given the financial constraints. Although the school had a focus on play, that was hard to do in an online class. I mirrored my phone on the TV so my son could have a larger image to look at. I know we have advantages over many grassroots families. We have lots of resources and enough space at home for my son to run around, which he needed because we couldn't really go out.

'When school switched to in-person classes, a student in my son's class got COVID. All 30 students as well as their parents, siblings, teachers, and their families were sent to Penny's Bay. The quarantine camp was newly opened, and it was chaotic; the government was still figuring out how to run it. The children who were in the same class as the infected students had to be quarantined for 21 days with a parent, but the other family members could leave after four days. I went in one room with our daughter, who was six months old, and my husband and son quarantined in the room next door. I was with Jasmine 24/7 and did all the diaper changing and feeding and FaceTimed with my son and husband next door. It was intense. Every night we were permitted to open the door to put out the garbage. Because we had rooms next to each other, we could say hello for two minutes before we had to shut the door. My son was upset in the beginning because he loves his sister and me and wanted us to be together, but we had scheduled FaceTime and there was boot camp to keep him busy and he adapted quickly. My husband said those weeks in Penny's Bay were memorable for him. He is usually at work and doesn't have that kind of intense time with our son. They slept together, ate together, did everything together. My husband said it helped him bond with our son and create a lasting memory. That quarantine experience has even given him the idea to do a solo boys' trip with our son every year, to make that special father-son time a regular thing.

'When I look back on that time, I realise that if not for the quarantine, the parents in my son's class wouldn't be as close as we are. We have a strong bond. The parents' WhatsApp chat group went crazy with everyone helping out with resources and materials. Parents were asking each other, do you have enough bed sheets, do you have enough food, because the food wasn't good. The teachers couldn't offer online classes because they were quarantined as well and had their families to take care of, so some of the school alumni stepped in. They sent us a schedule; it was like a boot camp, someone doing a music session, others offering story telling sessions. The PTA sent us resource packages and toys and snacks. In the end, because no one actually got COVID, they released everyone after two weeks.

'I clearly see a silver lining to the pandemic. I think faith plays a part in that. I believe everything is within God's control. We try to see the good side of things even when times are hard, and we try to teach this to our kids. We see the good in humanity.'

***Marie** (not her real name), a French national who has been teaching kindergarten and reception-year students at an international school for 15 years, was promoted to department head in 2018 in recognition of her hard work and dedication to her students. Despite the challenges posed by the pandemic, she found it to be a unique opportunity for self-reflection, personal growth, and a new direction.*

'In February 2020, I was on holiday with a friend when I got a message that the school would remain closed for another four days because of a virus. We were used to the school closing for a week or so during the social unrest or because of flu outbreaks, so we weren't especially worried. We were glad for the extra holiday. We never expected it to last three years.

'The pandemic arrived at a good time for me. I'd been in charge of my department for four years. In the beginning, I enjoyed the extra responsibility, but by 2020 I was working a lot and getting a bit fed up. At the beginning of the pandemic, we teachers had to go to school, but there were no students. We made videos for the kids and received what the parents sent back to us. We weren't yet teaching online, but we were producing content. It was a change of mindset which I found interesting. I had more time to spend with my colleagues and bond with them. It was a great year. The parents were very involved and impressed with the work we did even though the kids were not in class.

'When you teach you don't have time to think; you are always surrounded by people asking questions. You never have the time to follow an idea through to the end. That break from the crazy workday rhythm gave me the chance to withdraw and think. I had enjoyed being department head, but I didn't want to do it anymore. I realised I was close to burnout. I hadn't even recognised it as that because I was always on. That change of pace allowed me to recognise that the pressure had been too much. I had a chance to think about what I wanted to do and how I wanted to do it. If not for COVID, I probably would have renewed my contract without thinking about it. Instead, I had a chance to reflect, and I told the school that I wanted to step down as department head.

'In 2021, we taught the kids online, and sometimes they were in school. For kindergarten, we split the class into six groups of six and taught the same 15-minute lesson to each group. They each had a chance to speak, and we gave them something to prepare for the next day. For reception year, the online class was one hour. For two years we didn't have a full year in school with the kids. For the children, I wouldn't say it was a good time for them. It would have been better for them to be in school rather than learning online. But I appreciated the change. Working online, we had to rethink what we were doing and how we would work as a team. We shared a lot and got more organised. When we eventually went back into the classroom, we had a good system in place that we hadn't had before.

'A lot of the time, I didn't need to go into school and could prepare my online lessons at home. I live in a village on Lamma Island. Not having to commute saved me two hours a day. My friends were also working from home, and we'd meet in the village for lunch. I'd go back home and work in the afternoon and then meet friends for dinner. It was a relaxed pace of life.

'Now I had time to do something for myself that was nourishing. I signed up to do a hypnotherapy course. When you learn a therapy you also go through your own therapy, which I found very powerful. So, the pandemic was a double victory for me—I got a hypnotherapy qualification, and my own mental health improved. It felt good to develop a new skill outside my job.

'Hong Kong was quieter during COVID. Usually it's a 24-hour city, but the restrictions meant things closed at 6 pm. It was more like France, where things close early, and people go home to their family. It changed people. They had more time and were looking to make real connections instead of going out and getting crazy. I think it made everyone calm down a bit. I had a chance to think about who my real friends were and to make new connections. The quiet time was good for me.

'When we returned to school after COVID, everything was crazy again. Had we learned nothing from those two years? Before, my thinking had been very binary—should I stay, or should I leave? But then I thought of another possibility—to stay and work less. I asked if I could go from five days to four days a week, and the school agreed. It's a good balance for me and gives me the luxury of time. The pandemic gave me the chance to think about what is important to me in life. I had the time to think and readjust how I spend my time. I was lucky to keep my job and my salary. I'm happy to earn a little less money and have a more balanced life.'

***Aicha** (not her real name), a 31-year-old fashion designer, was born and raised in Israel. After serving two years in the military and completing four years at university, she arrived in Hong Kong as a fresh graduate. Despite missing her friends and family back home, Aicha credits the pandemic with creating the space for her to form a deep bond with her boyfriend and friendships that feel as close as family.*

'At the beginning of the pandemic I was quite new to Hong Kong and living on my own in a small apartment in Sai Ying Pun. Aside from the few friends who came with me from Israel to Hong Kong, I didn't know that many people. Then I met a friend who is very social, and he introduced me to his friends. They were an interesting mix, and that burst of meeting a whole lot of people who I could connect to felt huge. Soon after that, I met my boyfriend, Andre, through friends.

'COVID was very fresh and no one really knew what was going on; we'd only just started wearing masks. Andre and I ended up spending lots of time together, and the relationship got intense quickly. Our first conversations weren't the usual casual early relationship chats. We were talking about intense things, like family and the people we missed and the things we missed doing.

'The COVID regulations meant you could only dine out in small groups, so Andre and I ended up spending a lot of time one on one, which was a good thing for us to dive deep into the relationship. When you are going through hard emotional times, I think you get a better picture of who someone is, and if they are there for you.

'Andre was practically living in my apartment. My apartment was small, and it ended up being cramped, so we moved into a place together. In a normal relationship, you wouldn't move in after just six months of dating, but there was an intensity to the relationship because of the pandemic, and I felt comfortable enough to do that. The pandemic definitely accelerated our relationship. I'm sure that he's the right person for me, but I don't know if we would have stayed together if not for the pandemic. If not for COVID, we wouldn't have spent so much time together. I wouldn't have got to know him so quickly, which might have led to us breaking it off. In non-pandemic times there are so many distractions—online dating apps, busy bars, and clubs, travelling. There was none of that during the pandemic, and it slowed things down.

'It took a long time for me to accept the fact of quarantine, and I didn't travel for almost two years. Being stuck in Hong Kong and unable to visit family for quite a while meant I got really close to our friendship group. None of us were travelling; we were all in Hong Kong and went to each other's places. We were hanging out almost every day. Inevitably, you get attached to people quite quickly that way. We really connected, and they ended up being my family in Hong Kong.

'People elsewhere in the world might say they had the pandemic worse because they experienced full lockdown, but they had it over a short time. Although we weren't locked up, the rules were in place for three years. The friendship group really helped with the stress of not being able to leave and come back to Hong Kong.

'I do yoga almost every day. I got stressed when the yoga studios kept having to close, and then they brought out the rule that you had to wear a mask in class. I ended up doing a lot of classes online at home, where I didn't need to wear a mask. I knew it was important for me to keep doing yoga, so I didn't go down a path of being depressed and not in shape. I forced myself to do it, even when I was in that tiny apartment. I made it a daily routine to move a bit because I know I feel so much better when I do.

'I had been thinking about getting a tattoo for about 10 years, but I wasn't sure what I wanted, and was scared I would regret what I got or wouldn't like it. But I took the plunge during the pandemic. I think all the uncertainty, and the fact there were hard things happening in life, opened up a window for me to live more in the moment. I just decided to do it and got a tattoo of a flower on my back. Later, I got another on my arm.

'A lot of good things came to me during COVID. I might not have made this connection with Andre or made such close friendships if not for the pandemic. I also think I matured a lot in my personal development. I probably would have anyway, but it speeded up the process. I've enjoyed reflecting on those three years. It has helped me recognise the positive things that happened during COVID.'

* * *

As the pandemic swept across the globe, it brought with it a new way of life. Social distancing became the norm, and for many, this meant turning inward. It was a time of introspection and self-discovery as we grappled with the reality of our new existence. But as we navigated this uncharted territory, something unexpected happened. We began to appreciate the value of human connection. Separated from friends, colleagues, and loved ones, we realised that connection is a universal cure for mental health conditions.

The pandemic brought communities together in unexpected ways. A Facebook group called Hong Kong Quarantine Support Group was created in March 2020 to provide assistance and compassion to those in need. Within a year, the group had grown to nearly 30,000 members, many of whom had once been beneficiaries of the group's kindness. Even after their own needs were met, many members remained active in the group, offering support to others. By the time mandatory quarantine was lifted, the group had swelled to an impressive 97,000 members. This remarkable display of solidarity and compassion was a testament to the power of community in times of crisis.

Whether it's a brief interaction or a long Zoom call, moments when we feel connected to others can have a profound impact on our bodies. Our immune responses to stress are strengthened, oxytocin is released, and cardiovascular activity decreases. From a psychological perspective, these connections can act as a buffer against depression and bolster our mental health (Major et al., 2018).

One of the unexpected upsides of the pandemic was the shift to remote work. No longer bound by geography, workers found themselves with more time and flexibility. Commutes vanished, and work-life balance improved for many. People were able to be more available for their families and friends while still getting their work done. This period of enforced slowdown allowed some to reflect on how they spend their time and to consider what parts of this 'new normal' they wanted to maintain in the future.

The mandatory three-week quarantine, as discussed in an earlier chapter, presented many challenges. Yet, not all found it to be a negative experience, and there were those who struggled with it but also experienced some upsides. Judith Blaine's 2021 study on the impact of the Hong Kong quarantine on mental health revealed that some individuals found the isolation period to be an opportunity for self-reflection and growth. They slowed down, enjoyed their own company, and completed tasks. Some exercised more, while others learned new skills or picked up new hobbies. One individual used the 21-day quarantine to quit smoking; another focused on her studies. A woman shared how her husband connected more closely with their children due to the restrictions, and another enjoyed the less frantic pace of life. Many developed a deeper appreciation for fresh air, friends, family, and freedom. The most common positive to emerge was the support and kindness of strangers from the Hong Kong Quarantine Support Group.

The COVID-19 years brought with them a tumultuous upheaval, but amidst the chaos, an unexpected silver lining emerged: a shift in the way we view mental health challenges. It became clear that anyone could struggle with anxiety and depression under the right circumstances. These issues were widespread, and if you didn't experience them yourself, someone close to you likely did. While the stigma about mental health is far from gone in Hong Kong, the pandemic has opened a window for conversation. Discussions about mental health are now more common, and the government has pledged to make it a priority. The impact of stress and trauma on mental well-being is now a little better understood, and there is a greater awareness of the importance of addressing these issues.

Research indicates that positive psychology plays a crucial role in helping individuals overcome adversity. By engaging in reflective thinking and actively seeking the silver lining in difficult situations, we increase our chances of personal growth. The act of identifying benefits helps us recognise the protective factors in our lives, such as having strong relationships with family or friends, or own skills or strengths that can help us cope with stress more effectively. These factors serve as psychological buffers, shielding us from the potential harm of adverse situations (Waters et al., 2022).

Individuals who find greater meaning in their lives tend to experience higher levels of happiness, utilise their personal strengths more effectively, enjoy more fulfilling relationships, and are often perceived as more attractive potential friends. By learning techniques for positive reappraisal, individuals can find the silver lining in even the most difficult situations and focus on the things for which they are grateful. Gratitude can open the door to a new perspective on the world, allowing for personal growth and positive life changes even during times of crisis.

The COVID-19 pandemic has had a profound impact on our lives, bringing both challenges and opportunities for growth. While many have faced adversity, some have also experienced post-traumatic growth, a phenomenon where individuals undergo positive transformation following a traumatic event. This can manifest as changes in self-perception, relationships, and life philosophy. As such, the pandemic has presented opportunities for personal and societal transformation.

Strategies and Support

Positive reappraisal is a powerful tool that can help us find new meaning in challenging situations. By consciously focusing on the positive aspects of a situation, we can uncover opportunities for growth and personal development that may have been overlooked. This reframing allows us to find valuable learning experiences in challenges and opportunities for personal development in setbacks. Finding something to be grateful about in the face of adversity is a type of positive reappraisal.

Gratitude is a powerful force that can change the way we see the world. It is more than just saying 'thank you'. It's a powerful tool that can improve mental health, increase happiness, and help people cope with adversity. It is a habit of focusing on the positive aspects of daily life, allowing us to interpret negative events in a more fruitful way. When we are grateful, anxiety, depression, and negativism are limited. We are able to appreciate the many good things the world offers and bestows upon us. Gratitude changes our perspective, reorienting our attention towards others and the world beyond ourselves.

Research shows that practising gratitude can reduce negative emotions like anxiety and depression, while boosting positive feelings and overall life satisfaction. And during tough times, like a pandemic, gratitude can be a lifeline. Studies have found that gratitude interventions helped people feel less afraid of COVID-19, less stressed, and more connected to others (Kumar et al., 2022).

Of course, no amount of gratitude can undo the systemic inequalities that have been highlighted and exacerbated by the pandemic. But practising gratitude may provide at least some temporary relief from the negative effects of COVID-19 and other adverse situations.

Practising gratitude in your daily life can be easy and effective. Here are some simple methods to cultivate gratitude:

Gratitude Journaling: Take a few minutes each day to write down five things you are grateful for. It could be something as simple as a kind gesture from a friend, a delicious meal, or a beautiful sunset. Doing this before bed is a great way to end the day on a positive and thankful note.

Express Gratitude to Others: Make time to express gratitude to the people in your life. Whether it's a quick thank-you to a colleague or a heartfelt message to a friend, acknowledging the kindness of others will uplift both you and the receiver.

Gratitude Walks: Take a walk in nature and focus your attention on the things you appreciate. It could be having supportive friends or the fact you and your loved ones are in good health. Once you feel gratitude in your heart, pay attention to the beauty around you. Notice the colours of the leaves, the sound of birdsong, and the smells of the natural world. Express gratitude for the wonders of nature. When we think of the things we are grateful for, it is natural to think of the big experiences in our lives, such as friends, family, job, and health. These are certainly important, but it's also important to appreciate the simple everyday pleasures that often go unnoticed: a hug from a child, sharing a joke with a friend, or the freshness of the first day of autumn after the long hot summer.

14

Ways Forward

Access to Mental Health

In the face of adversity, Hong Kong has proven time and time again to be a resilient city. It always bounces back. As we emerge from the shadow of the pandemic, it is only natural for people to be eager to move forward. However, to do so without reflecting on the lessons learned would be a missed opportunity. Another pandemic is inevitable—it's not a question of if but when. As such, preparation for such an event should be treated as an ongoing priority. The insights gained from our recent experience with COVID-19 can and must inform our response to the next pandemic.

During the pandemic, Hong Kong, like the rest of the world, saw a surge in rates of anxiety and depression. The lifting of the mask mandate in March 2023 may have marked the official end of the pandemic, but mental health issues continued to rise. In the wake of a brutal stabbing in a shopping centre that claimed the lives of two women, the government acknowledged the need for enhanced mental health support. In a meeting in June 2023, the government's Advisory Committee on Mental Health recommended action in 10 areas. However, many of these recommendations echoed those made in a 2017 independent review of the city's mental health policies. On critical issues such as human resources, the committee had little to say. Now is the time for an open review, acting on recommendations and investing in mental health in Hong Kong.

The people who shared their experiences of the pandemic for this book did so with a purpose. Speaking frankly and openly about deeply personal matters, they hope to ensure that when the next pandemic strikes, we are better informed and better prepared. Their first-hand accounts provide valuable insights into how we can learn from the experience of COVID-19. Guided by their lived experiences, this concluding chapter explores six key areas: Anti-stigma, Communication, Compassion, Education, Social Vulnerability, and Support. By adopting the acronym 'ACCESS', we can envision a path towards improved access to mental health resources and better mental well-being in the face of the next pandemic.

Anti-stigma

The risk of facing discrimination in cultural, social, and professional spheres creates a formidable barrier to seeking treatment for mental health issues. People may fear being shunned by family and friends or that disclosing a mental health condition could jeopardise their career prospects or cost them their job. Personal beliefs about mental illness can also prevent people from acknowledging their condition, seeking help, or adhering to treatment.

In Chapter 6, Dr Chan bravely revealed the struggles he faced in seeking support for his mental health. His fear of being perceived as weak, and the negative attitudes he witnessed among his colleagues towards those who sought help, made him hesitant to seek counselling from his employer. Similarly, Tom, a nurse who also shared his experience in Chapter 6, found himself discouraged from attending a workshop on psychological support for frontline staff. Despite the workshop being offered by his hospital, Tom was deterred by the disparaging remarks made by his superiors about a colleague who had been open about their mental health struggles.

The cultural aspect of stigma cannot be overlooked. In Chapter 9, Catalina, a Filipina domestic helper, explained that within the migrant worker community, there is a reluctance to openly discuss mental health. To do so risks being perceived as weak and becoming the subject of gossip and raises concerns that stories may even reach their friends and family back in the Philippines. There is also a fear that it could jeopardise their employment.

In Cantonese and among Hong Kong's minority communities, it is all too common to hear name-calling and shaming with words like 'mad', 'crazy', and 'attention-seeker'. But we can effect positive change right now by committing to think carefully about the words we use and the impact they have. A first step is accepting that we are all vulnerable to the stresses of daily life—especially so in a pandemic—and understanding that recovery is possible. Just as we can recover from other illnesses or injuries, so too can we recover from mental health problems.

While the stigmas about mental health are deeply ingrained and won't disappear overnight, there is hope. Through awareness and education campaigns, we can work to change public perceptions and break down the barriers to treatment. In 2023, a study by Mind HK found that stigma and discrimination against those with mental health conditions had worsened during the pandemic. It was thought that the messaging about the need to isolate from the sick had been translated into mental health as well. In response, Mind HK launched a month-long anti-stigma campaign called #HonestlySpeaking in

August 2023. With more than 100 ambassadors sharing their mental health struggles, the campaign aimed to challenge misconceptions and encourage open and honest conversations about mental health. Initiatives like this help to chip away at the stigma and create a more supportive and inclusive society.

Communication

The importance of clear and timely communication cannot be overstated. Having access to accurate and transparent information is essential in managing the fear, anxiety, and panic that can take hold during a pandemic. Technology-based information-exchange platforms can play a crucial role in facilitating this.

In Chapter 2, Siu-hang, who was 22 weeks pregnant when she was sent to Penny's Bay quarantine camp, shared her experience. She said that if she had been able to speak to a human during her isolation, her fears wouldn't have escalated like they did. Similarly, new mother Monique, mentioned in Chapter 5, said that clearer communication and explanation about what was happening would have greatly reduced her stress. For her, the hardest part of the pandemic was not knowing what was happening. She believes that the uncertainty could have been better managed if there was one place where current regulations and information were posted so that everyone—parents, doctors, and nurses—could be on the same page and informed. Bobo, a nurse who served on the COVID wards through the pandemic, shared her story in Chapter 6. She said her stress came not from the virus but from constantly changing guidelines. She too said that more consistent and clearer guidelines would have reduced a lot of anxiety.

As some older adults mainly receive information from free-to-air TV, it is important to ensure that they are kept well informed. One solution could be to have a TV channel devoted to the pandemic. However, instead of merely delivering an endless replay of pandemic press briefings, this platform should make news and information accessible, engaging, and uplifting for viewers.

Aaron Busch, better known by his Twitter (now known as X) handle Tripperhead, became Hong Kong's unofficial spokesperson for all things COVID-19. For 1,036 consecutive days, he deciphered government press releases and crunched COVID-19 figures, making the official data accessible (Whitehead, 2023). His efforts were greatly appreciated, and his 51,000 Twitter followers were testament to the demand for comprehensive information and a platform where they could ask urgent questions and receive support. Similarly, the Hong Kong Quarantine Support Group, a Facebook community, played a crucial role in helping many people feel included by offering crowd-sourced advice, up-to-date information, and a sympathetic ear.

Community

In times of crisis, such as a pandemic, the bonds of community become our lifeline. Recent research by Im and Sim (2023) has shown that cultivating a positive sense of community can alleviate negative responses to the pandemic, such as depression and anxiety, and promote growth. By being considerate and helpful towards those in our community, we can foster strong interpersonal relationships, leading to deep friendships and a willingness to accept help from others. When we face challenges together, a sense of community allows us to view our struggles from a broader perspective, transcending personal concerns.

In Chapter 2, Kelvin recounts his experience of being under compulsory lockdown at his home on the Kwai Chung Estate. Despite feeling isolated from the outside world, Kelvin and his family found solace in the support of their neighbours. United by their shared circumstances, they saw themselves as being 'in the same boat' and their bond with nearby families grew stronger. During this trying time, they shared information and resources, drawing closer together as a community. The strength of their connections with their neighbours helped them navigate a stressful experience.

In Chapter 10, Ma Jeuk echoes a similar sentiment, expressing her appreciation for the psychological support provided by her small but strong network of friends and family living nearby. They shared food and resources, but it was the emotional support of this tight-knit community that proved most valuable.

With a sense of community and the understanding that we are all in this together, compassion naturally arises. We no longer see our neighbours or those around us as 'other': We are all humans going through a shared experience. Small gestures of kindness can have a profound impact, bolstering resilience and helping us navigate uncertain times. The beauty of kindness is that it benefits both the giver and the receiver, providing a positive psychological gain for all involved.

Kindness and compassion need not be grand gestures—they can be as simple as a smile or a few words of encouragement. In Chapter 7, Laura Hazlett shares how the kindness of a nurse helped her manage the devastation of being separated from her daughter. Though the nurse could not change the facts of the situation, her empathy and compassion changed Laura's outlook. In times of hardship, small acts of kindness can ripple through a community, providing comfort and support to those in need.

During a crisis, we can connect with our own immediate communities. Whether it be through small acts of kindness towards our neighbours, colleagues, and friends, or connecting with the less fortunate through NGOs or charities, we all have a role to play in strengthening our communities. Governments, schools, and universities can lead by example, promoting the values of social cooperation and responsibility through targeted campaigns. In coming together, we can safeguard the lives and freedoms of individuals and ensure that we are all better prepared to face the next pandemic.

Education

In the midst of the pandemic, fear was an ever-present companion. A study conducted in the first year surveyed 2,822 adults in Hong Kong and mainland China, revealing that more than 40 percent reported feeling scared by the thought of COVID-19 (Choi et al., 2022). The fear of infection loomed large, compounded by concerns that the health care system would be overwhelmed by the rising number of cases. For many, memories of the 2003 SARS epidemic resurfaced, intensifying their fears. As Samantha notes in Chapter 5, fear was pervasive. She reflects that it would have been more productive to approach COVID-19 as an illness to be treated rather than as something to be feared.

Fear is the embodiment of the unknown, the unthinkable, and the worst-case scenario. Yet, there is an antidote to this anxiety and fear: understanding, brought about by knowledge. With knowledge, the unknown becomes known, and the worst-case scenario becomes an extremely unlikely event. When armed with knowledge of why and how, the sting of anxiety and fear can be tempered. As we saw in

Chapter 5, expectant mothers who were equipped with knowledge on how to prevent COVID-19 infection were less fearful of the virus.

In Chapter 10, Winnie Cheung recounts her experience of spending hours poring over the news online, only to be left feeling anxious and overwhelmed by the constantly shifting narrative. Wary of which news sources to trust, she eventually stopped following the news and delayed getting vaccinated. Cheung reflects that more accessible information and better education about the virus and vaccines would have helped to ease her fears.

More and better education also leads to compassion and kindness. As Ms Li notes in Chapter 10, if more people have a deeper understanding of the challenges faced by those undertaking unpredictable quarantines, they are more likely to be empathetic. An appreciation of what she was going through from those far away would have helped her better cope with her isolation.

In an age when social media has given rise to a cacophony of voices, all vying for attention, it is essential that we educate people with the skills and knowledge to identify fake or inaccurate news. Knowing what a trusted news source looks like and when information is unreliable is crucial in preventing the spread of misinformation and the panic that often ensues. By empowering people with the ability to discern fact from fiction, we can promote a more informed and rational discourse.

Social Vulnerability

The pandemic exposed the stark reality of life for Hong Kong's most marginalised communities, revealing deep-seated inequalities in the city. Vulnerable groups such as low-income residents, women, elderly people, and minorities were hit hardest by the crisis, their vulnerabilities intensified by limited access to resources and facilities. Social vulnerability—the harm inflicted on these groups due to their limited access to services—was particularly pronounced among these populations.

In June 2023, just a few months after the lifting of the mask mandate, a tragedy struck in Sham Shui Po, a working-class neighbourhood. A mother was charged with murdering her three young daughters in their 200-square-foot subdivided flat. This heartbreaking incident speaks to the lack of support for non-Chinese-speaking ethnic minority groups.

The mental strain of social isolation is a burden borne by all, but it weighs heaviest on those with limited resources, confined to cramped living spaces. Kelvin, a resident of a public housing estate that endured a seven-day lockdown in January 2022, knows this all too well. In Chapter 2, he shared that maintaining mental health during lockdown hinges on having enough personal space. When he opened his window, he heard his neighbours shouting and cursing at each other, crumbling under the pressure of so many family members confined in a tiny 300-square-foot flat.

Ma Jeuk, who comes from a working-class family and lives in a small flat with her husband and parents, shared her story in Chapter 10. She expressed her frustration at the stark contrast between the lives of the rich and the poor, which she said was only magnified by the pandemic. After the lifting of the mask mandate, she noticed people in the affluent Central district taking off their masks. She said many people in her working-class neighbourhood continued to wear masks because they couldn't afford to get sick and miss work.

In Chapter 3, primary schoolteacher Winter shared her observations about the effect of the pandemic on education. She said that the gap between the children from lower-income families and those from more privileged families had widened during the pandemic. Children from working-class families were limited in their social connection with peers and teachers due to inadequate digital devices and poor internet access. While better-off parents with more resources were able to help their children catch up on missed schooling, those from low-income families had fallen even further behind.

To enhance our resilience against future pandemics, it is crucial that we prioritise reducing inequalities. Improving the accessibility of services and facilities for the vulnerable during times of crisis is essential. By doing so, we can contribute to better recovery capacities, helping communities to bounce back more quickly from the impact of a pandemic.

Support / Mental Health

The ongoing struggle to meet the mental health needs of patients and their families is exacerbated by a chronic shortage of qualified staff. A comprehensive review of mental health policies is urgently needed, its findings made public and funds allocated for action to be taken. This issue will not resolve itself—it demands immediate attention and resources. The longer it is neglected, the more dire the situation will become. It is time for decisive action to address this pressing concern.

In addition to the general public, frontline health care workers—including doctors, nurses, and staff in elderly care homes—urgently require psychological support. They have been at the forefront of the pandemic, bearing the brunt of its effect. It is essential that we maintain a psychologically healthy workforce, not only for their well-being but also for the sustainability of our health care system. Failure to support them may result in even more doctors and nurses leaving the public system, further exacerbating the current shortage of qualified staff.

In Chapter 6, Dr Lam highlights the need for change within the health care system, citing a toxic work environment that stigmatises those seeking mental health support. She advocates for a shift away from a hierarchical culture in hospitals towards one that fosters team collaboration and diversity. There are people within the system who are ready and willing to embrace this change, and it is imperative that their voices be heard and their efforts supported.

Local NGOs are making a significant impact in addressing mental health needs. Mind HK, for example, offers excellent online resources and provided short-term, pro bono mental health support during the first year of the pandemic. ImpactHK supports the homeless with accommodation, training, and counselling. The HELP for Domestic Workers' MeHeal programme offers free counselling for migrant workers. However, as noted by Miriam (Chapter 9) and Tai Lui (Chapter 11), many people are unaware of these free services, which can be life-saving. The government has a responsibility to work with these organisations to raise awareness and ensure that those in need have access to the support they require. During a pandemic, it is more important than ever for the government to collaborate with community resources rather than attempting to do everything by itself.

It is essential to address the barriers that prevent people from accessing available support. In Chapter 8, pilot John discussed the double-edged sword of seeking help from his employer. Despite recognising his need for support, he refrained from asking, for fear of jeopardising his job security and future prospects. Trapped within the closed-loop system for more than two years, John and his colleagues were subjected to immense psychological pressure. They recognised this as an unspoken safety issue, one that demanded attention. It is of utmost importance to foster an environment where people feel secure and supported in seeking the help they need.

* * *

This book is a testament to the resilience and determination of those who have lived through the pandemic in Hong Kong and a reminder of the importance of coming together to support one another in times of need. It is a powerful call to action, urging us to learn from the past and work towards a better future.

For policymakers, the personal accounts contained within these pages offer invaluable insights into the challenges faced during the pandemic and can help inform future policy decisions. But this book is more than just a tool for policymakers; it is also a means for people to process their own experiences of the pandemic. By seeing their struggles acknowledged and named in print, and by recognising that they are part of a collective suffering, readers can take a step towards healing. The strategies suggested at the end of each chapter offer practical advice for bolstering mental health. Just as we strive to maintain good physical health through diet and exercise, so too can we take proactive steps to safeguard our mental health. We do not need to wait for the next pandemic to prioritise our mental well-being.

Works Cited

Abrams, L. (2013, January 22). When trees die, people die. *The Atlantic*. https://www.theatlantic.com/health/archive/2013/01/when-trees-die-people-die/267322/

Billings, J., Ching, B. C. F., Gkofa, V., Greene, T., & Bloomfield, M. (2021). Experiences of frontline healthcare workers and their views about support during COVID-19 and previous pandemics: A systematic review and qualitative meta-synthesis. *BMC Health Services Research*, *21*, 1–17.

Blaine, J. (2021). Exploring the psychosocial consequences of mandatory quarantine during the COVID-19 pandemic in Hong Kong. *Psychology and Behavioral Sciences*, *10*(2), 96–103.

Blaine, J. (2022). Teachers' mental wellbeing during ongoing school closures in Hong Kong. *Education Journal*, *11*(4), 143–156.

Bratman, G. N., Anderson, C. B., Berman, M. G., Cochran, B., De Vries, S., Flanders, J., . . . & Daily, G. C. (2019). Nature and mental health: An ecosystem service perspective. *Science Advances*, *5*(7), eaax0903.

Brooks, S. K., Webster, R. K., Smith, L. E., Woodland, L., Wessely, S., Greenberg, N., & Rubin, G. J. (2020). The psychological impact of quarantine and how to reduce it: Rapid review of the evidence. *The Lancet*, *395*(10227), 912–920.

Bohren, M. A., Hofmeyr, G. J., Sakala, C., Fukuzawa, R. K., & Cuthbert, A. (2017). Continuous support for women during childbirth. *Cochrane Database of Systematic Reviews*, (7). Art. No.: CD003766. https://doi.org/10.1002/14651858.CD003766.pub6

Cahill, J., Cullen, P., & Gaynor, K. (2022). The case for change: Aviation worker wellbeing during the COVID 19 pandemic, and the need for an integrated health and safety culture. *Cognition, Technology & Work*, 1–43.

Carnay, N. (2017). *Investigating living accommodation of women domestic migrant workers towards advocacy and action*. Mission For Migrant Workers. https://www.ohchr.org/sites/default/files/Documents/Issues/Migration/CFI-COVID/SubmissionsCOVID/CSO/Pictures.pdf

Catalano, G., Houston, S. H., Catalano, M. C., Butera, A. S., Jennings, S. M., Hakala, S. M., . . . & Laliotis, G. J. (2003). Anxiety and depression in hospitalized patients in resistant organism isolation. *Southern Medical Journal*, *96*(2), 141–146.

Chan, F., Kapai, P., & Wisniewski, O. (2022, March 20). More humane policies would not leave pregnant women in Hong Kong dreading delivery or worried about being separated from their children [Letter to the editor]. *South China Morning Post*, https://www.scmp.com/comment/letters/article/3170814/more-humane-policies-would-not-leave-pregnant-women-hong-kong

Chan, H., & Riordan, P. (2022, November 12). Cathay's pilot exodus persists as pandemic curbs hit morale. *Financial Times*. https://www.ft.com/content/c906a883-94ad-438a-974d-fb8c42ce448c

Chau, C. (2023, January 29). "The frontline in our homes": Covid-19's lasting impact on Hong Kong's migrant domestic workers. *Hong Kong Free Press*. https://hongkongfp.com/2023/01/29/the-frontline-in-our-homes-covid-19s-lasting-impact-on-hong-kongs-migrant-domestic-workers/

Cheng, C., Wong, W. M., & Tsang, K. W. (2006). Perception of benefits and costs during SARS outbreak: An 18-month prospective study. *Journal of Consulting and Clinical Psychology*, *74*(5), 870.

Cheung, A. T., Ho, L. L. K., Li, W. H. C., Chung, J. O. K., & Smith, G. D. (2023). Psychological distress experienced by nurses amid the fifth wave of the COVID-19 pandemic in Hong Kong: A qualitative study. *Frontiers in Public Health*, *10*, 1023302.

Cheung, T., & Yip, P. S. (2015). Depression, anxiety and symptoms of stress among Hong Kong nurses: A cross-sectional study. *International Journal of Environmental Research and Public Health*, *12*(9), 11072–11100.

Choi, E. P., Duan, W., Fong, D. Y., Lok, K. Y., Ho, M., Wong, J. Y., & Lin, C. C. (2022). Psychometric evaluation of a fear of COVID-19 scale in China: Cross-sectional study. *JMIR Formative Research*, *6*(3), e31992.

Chung, R. Y. N., & Mak, J. K. L. (2020). Physical and mental health of live-in female migrant domestic workers: A randomly sampled survey in Hong Kong. *American Behavioral Scientist*, *64*(6), 802–822.

Chinese University of Hong Kong. (2022, June). COVID-19 pandemic disrupted the daily lives of schoolchildren in Hong Kong. https://www.med.cuhk.edu.hk/press-releases/covid-pandemic-disrupted-the-daily-life-of-schoolchildren-in-hong-kong-the-proportion-of-overweight-and-obese-kids-more-than-doubled

City University Hong Kong. (2021, October 6). Physical and mental health of socially isolated seniors at higher risk during pandemic. https://www.cb.cityu.edu.hk/News-and-Events/news/2021/10/Physical-and-mental-health-socially-isolated-seniors-higher-risk-during-pandemic

Das, M. (2022). COVID-19 and the elderlies: How safe are Hong Kong's care homes? *Frontiers in Public Health*, 10, 883472.

Dinibutun, S. R. (2020). Factors associated with burnout among physicians: An evaluation during a period of COVID-19 pandemic. *Journal of Healthcare Leadership*, 85–94.

Fan, H. S. L., Choi, E. P. H., Ko, R. W. T., Kwok, J. Y. Y., Wong, J. Y. H., Fong, D. Y. T., . . . & Lok, K. Y. W. (2022). COVID-19 related fear and depression of pregnant women and new mothers. *Public Health Nursing*, *39*(3), 562–571.

Fransson, E., Örtenstrand, A., & Hjelmstedt, A. (2011). Antenatal depressive symptoms and preterm birth: A prospective study of a Swedish national sample. *Birth*, *38*(1), 10–16.

Freed, J. (2021, November 21). Locked in: Hong Kong COVID rules take mental toll on Cathay pilots. *Reuters*. https://www.reuters.com/world/asia-pacific/locked-hotels-hong-kongs-covid-19-rules-take-mental-toll-cathay-pilots-2021-11-26/

Goodman, M. J., & Schorling, J. B. (2012). A mindfulness course decreases burnout and improves well-being among healthcare providers. *The International Journal of Psychiatry in Medicine, 43(2), 119–128.*

Hansen, M. M., Jones, R., & Tocchini, K. (2017). Shinrin-yoku (forest bathing) and nature therapy: A state-of-the-art review. *International Journal of Environmental Research and Public Health*, *14*(8), 851.

Hawryluck, L., Gold, W. L., Robinson, S., Pogorski, S., Galea, S., & Styra, R. (2004). SARS control and psychological effects of quarantine, Toronto, Canada. *Emerging Infectious Diseases*, *10*(7), 1206.

Hazan, H., & Chan, C. S. (2022). Indirect contact with nature, lifestyle, and mental health outcomes during mandatory hotel quarantine in Hong Kong. *Journal of Mental Health*, 1–7.

HelperChoice. (2022, August 23). 3 out of 10 domestic workers in urgent financial and emotional support in the fifth wave, employers rise up to support. https://www.helperchoice.com/c/press-centre/survey-3-out-of-10-domestic-workers-in-urgent-financial-and-emotional-support

Heung, S., & Lam, J. (2022, January 15). 'Quarantine is not punishment'. *South China Morning Post*. https://www.scmp.com/news/hong-kong/health-environment/article/3163512/quarantine-not-punishment-angry-residents-hong

Ho, K. H. M., & Smith, G. D. (2020). A discursive paper on the importance of health literacy among foreign domestic workers during outbreaks of communicable diseases. *Journal of Clinical Nursing*, *29*(23–24), 4827–4833.

Ho, K. H. M., Yang, C., Leung, A. K. Y., Bressington, D., Chien, W. T., Cheng, Q., & Cheung, D. S. K. (2022). Peer support and mental health of migrant domestic workers: A scoping review. *International Journal of Environmental Research and Public Health*, *19*(13), 7617.

Hong Kong Baptist University. (2022, March 31). *Understanding how to boost elderly vaccination rate*. https://research.hkbu.edu.hk/f/page/20923/23044/EN-COVID%20Report_Tsang_Final.pdf

Hornor G. (2015). Childhood trauma exposure and toxic stress: What the PNP needs to know. *Journal of Pediatric Health Care: Official Publication of National Association of Pediatric Nurse Associates & Practitioners*, *29*(2), 191–198. https://doi.org/10.1016/j.pedhc.2014.09.006

Howard, K., Martin, A., Berlin, L. J., & Brooks-Gunn, J. (2011). Early mother-child separation, parenting, and child well-being in Early Head Start families. *Attachment & Human Development*, *13*(1), 5–26. https://doi.org/10.1080/14616734.2010.488119

Hui, P. W., Seto, M. T., & Cheung, K. W. (2022). Behavioural adaptations and responses to obstetric care among pregnant women during an early stage of the COVID-19 pandemic in Hong Kong: A cross-sectional survey. *Hong Kong Medical Journal, 28*(5), 367.

Hung, E. (2023, May 12). More than 16 per cent of Hong Kong's young people have likely mental health issues, large-scale study finds. *South China Morning Post*. https://www.scmp.com/news/hong-kong/health-environment/article/3220259/more-16-cent-hong-kongs-young-people-have-likely-psychiatric-problem-large-scale-study-finds

Hunter, M. R., Gillespie, B. W., & Chen, S. Y. P. (2019). Urban nature experiences reduce stress in the context of daily life based on salivary biomarkers. *Frontiers in Psychology*, 722.

Im, S. Y., & Sim, J. C. (2023). The impact of COVID-19 pandemic on mental health and posttraumatic growth of Korean college students: A mixed method study examining the moderating role of coping flexibility and sense of community. *Frontiers in Psychology, 14*, 1200570.

Jans-Beken, L., Jacobs, N., Janssens, M., Peeters, S., Reijnders, J., Lechner, L., & Lataster, J. (2020). Gratitude and health: An updated review. *The Journal of Positive Psychology, 15*(6), 743–782.

Jeong, H., Yim, H. W., Song, Y. J., Ki, M., Min, J. A., Cho, J., & Chae, J. H. (2016). Mental health status of people isolated due to Middle East Respiratory Syndrome. *Epidemiology and Health, 38*.

Kumar, S. A., Edwards, M. E., Grandgenett, H. M., Scherer, L. L., DiLillo, D., & Jaffe, A. E. (2022). Does gratitude promote resilience during a pandemic? An examination of mental health and positivity at the onset of COVID-19. *Journal of Happiness Studies, 23*(7), 3463–3483.

Lam, N. (2021, October 5). Over 70 per cent of young doctors in Hong Kong burnt out from work, one-fifth have depression, survey shows. *South China Morning Post*. https://www.scmp.com/news/hong-kong/health-environment/article/3151290/over-70-cent-young-doctors-hong-kong-burnt-out

Lau, J. T., Yang, X., Tsui, H. Y., Pang, E., & Wing, Y. K. (2006). Positive mental health-related impacts of the SARS epidemic on the general public in Hong Kong and their associations with other negative impacts. *Journal of Infection, 53*(2), 114–124.

Leung, K. K. Y., & Hon, K. L. E. (2021). The role of media messaging in COVID-19 vaccine hesitancy amongst the student population: Friend or foe. *Pediatric Pulmonology, 56*(12), 4066.

Li, P. (2021, July 31). COVID-19 vaccination in elderly—Physician perspectives [Webinar]. Hong Kong College of Physicians. https://www.hkam.org.hk/sites/default/files/PDFs/COVID-19%20Vaccination%20in%20Elderly%20–%20Physician%20perspectives_by%20Prof%20Philip%20Li.pdf

Lok, W. Y., Chow, C. Y., Kong, C. W., & To, W. W. (2022). Knowledge, attitudes, and behaviours of pregnant women towards COVID-19: A cross-sectional survey. *Hong Kong Medical Journal, 28*(2), 124.

Lui, I. D., Vandan, N., Davies, S. E., Harman, S., Morgan, R., Smith, J., . . . & Grépin, K. A. (2021). "We also deserve help during the pandemic": The effect of the COVID-19 pandemic on foreign domestic workers in Hong Kong. *Journal of Migration and Health*, *3*, 100037.

Ma, J., (2022, March 9). More than half of Hong Kong workers lost income after testing positive for coronavirus, survey finds. *South China Morning Post*. https://www.scmp.com/news/hong-kong/health-environment/article/3169822/more-half-hong-kong-workers-lost-income-after

Major, B. C., Le Nguyen, K. D., Lundberg, K. B., & Fredrickson, B. L. (2018). Well-being correlates of perceived positivity resonance: Evidence from trait and episode-level assessments. *Personality and Social Psychology Bulletin*, *44*(12), 1631–1647.

Master, F., & Murdoch, S. (2022, September 11). COVID rules cast clouds over Hong Kong schools. *Reuters*. https://www.reuters.com/world/china/unrelenting-covid-rules-cast-clouds-over-hong-kong-schools-2022-09-11/

Maunder, R. G. (2009). Was SARS a mental health catastrophe? *General Hospital Psychiatry*, *31*(4), 316.

Mikkelsen, K., Stojanovska, L., Polenakovic, M., Bosevski, M., & Apostolopoulos, V. (2017). Exercise and mental health. *Maturitas*, *106*, 48–56.

Mind HK. (2022, April 7). *Mind HK survey reveals Hong Kong citizens' worsening state of mental health during the fifth wave of the Covid-19 pandemic* [Press release]. https://www.mind.org.hk/press-releases/mind-hk-survey-reveals-hong-kong-citizens-worsening-state-of-mental-health-during-the-fifth-wave-of-the-covid-19-pandemic/

Muramoto, M., Kita, S., Tobe, H., Ikeda, M., & Kamibeppu, K. (2022). The association between self-compassion in the postnatal period and difficult experiences with COVID-19 pandemic-related changes during pregnancy: An observational study for women at 1-month postnatal in Japan. *Japan Journal of Nursing Science*, *19*(4), e12494.

Pan, P. J., Chang, S. H., & Yu, Y. Y. (2005). A support group for home-quarantined college students exposed to SARS: Learning from practice. *The Journal for Specialists in Group Work*, *30*(4), 363–374.

Paul, E. (2021, March 23). 10 Hong Kong quarantine hacks to help you survive: Pack alcohol, snacks, candles, and a SIM card—there's no Wi-fi. *South China Morning Post*. https://www.scmp.com/lifestyle/health-wellness/article/3126529/10-quarantine-hacks-help-you-survive-hong-kongs-tough-14

The Samaritan Befrienders Hong Kong. (2022). *2021 Annual report of the Samaritan befrienders Hong Kong*. https://sbhk.org.hk/wp-content/uploads/2022/09/2021-Annual-Report.pdf

Save The Children. (2020, September). *Mental health matters*. https://savethechildren.org.hk/wp-content/uploads/2020/09/Mental-Health-Matters-Save-the-Children-Hong-Kong-2020.pdf

Schraedley, P. K., Turner, R. J., & Gotlib, I. H. (2002). Stability of retrospective reports in depression: Traumatic events, past depressive episodes, and parental psychopathology. *Journal of Health and Social Behavior, 43*(3), 307–316. https://doi.org/10.2307/3090206

Shah, A. S., Wood, R., Gribben, C., Caldwell, D., Bishop, J., Weir, A., . . . & McAllister, D. A. (2020). Risk of hospital admission with coronavirus disease 2019 in healthcare workers and their households: Nationwide linkage cohort study. *British Medical Journal, 371.*

Shonkoff, J. P., Garner, A. S., Committee on Psychosocial Aspects of Child and Family Health, Committee on Early Childhood, Adoption, and Dependent Care, & Section on Developmental and Behavioral Pediatrics (2012). The lifelong effects of early childhood adversity and toxic stress. *Pediatrics, 129*(1), e232–e246. https://doi.org/10.1542/peds.2011-2663

Stadler, K. (2022). The psychological impact of COVID-19 on pilot mental health and wellbeing—Quarantine experiences. *Transportation Research Procedia, 66*, 179–186.

Summers, J. K., & Vivian, D. N. (2018). Ecotherapy—A forgotten ecosystem service: A review. *Frontiers in Psychology, 9*, 1389.

Sun, F. (2022, March 29). Up to 2,000 children under age 10 separated from parents in Hong Kong hospitals over past 6 weeks after catching Covid-19. *South China Morning Post.* https://scmp.com/news/hong-kong/health-environment/article/3172180/2000-children-under-age-10-separated-parents-hong?

Taylor, L. (2022). Covid-19: Hong Kong reports world's highest death rate as zero covid strategy fails. *British Medical Journal, 376*(o420), 35177535.

The Samaritan Befrienders Hong Kong. (2022). *2021 annual report of the Samaritan befrienders Hong Kong.* https://sbhk.org.hk/wp-content/uploads/2022/09/2021-Annual-Report.pdf

Thompson, D. R., Lopez, V., Lee, D., & Twinn, S. (2004). SARS—A perspective from a school of nursing in Hong Kong. *Journal of Clinical Nursing, 13*(2), 131–135.

Tso, W. W. Y., Wong, R. S., Tung, K. T. S., Rao, N., Fu, K. W., Yam, J. C. S., Chua, G. T., Chen, E. Y. H., Lee, T. M. C., Chan, S. K. W., Wong, W. H. S., Xiong, X., Chui, C. S., Li, X., Wong, K., Leung, C., Tsang, S. K. M., Chan, G. C. F., Tam, P. K. H., Chan, K. L., . . . Lp, P. (2022). Vulnerability and resilience in children during the COVID-19 pandemic. *European Child & Adolescent Psychiatry, 31*(1), 161–176. https://doi.org/10.1007/s00787-020-01680-8

University of Hong Kong. (2022a, September 10). *Moving forward together* [Press release]. https://www.hku.hk/press/news_detail_25024.html

University of Hong Kong. (2022b, October 10) *Survey reveals over a third of older adults in Hong Kong suffered from emotional distress in the fifth wave of COVID-19* [Press release]. https://www.hku.hk/press/press-releases/detail/25189.html

University of Southern Australia. (2022, August 3). Pandemic has put long-haul pilots in a stressful tailspin. https://www.unisa.edu.au/media-centre/Releases/2022/pandemic-has-put-long-haul-pilots-in-a-stressful-tailspin/

Uplifters. (2020). Findings of a mental health need assessment survey for migrant domestic workers in Hong Kong. https://uplifters-edu.org/wp-content/uploads/

2021/04/A-Mental-Health-Need-Assessment-Survey-for-Migrant-Domestic-Workers-in-Hong-Kong.pdf

Van den Bergh, B. R., Mulder, E. J., Mennes, M., & Glover, V. (2005). Antenatal maternal anxiety and stress and the neurobehavioural development of the fetus and child: Links and possible mechanisms. A review. *Neuroscience & Biobehavioral Reviews, 29*(2), 237–258.

Wassenberg, M. W. M., Severs, D., & Bonten, M. J. M. (2010). Psychological impact of short-term isolation measures in hospitalised patients. *Journal of Hospital Infection, 75*(2), 124–127.

Waters, L., Algoe, S. B., Dutton, J., Emmons, R., Fredrickson, B. L., Heaphy, E., . . . & Steger, M. (2022). Positive psychology in a pandemic: Buffering, bolstering, and building mental health. *The Journal of Positive Psychology, 17*(3), 303–323.

Westbrook, L. (2022, February 20). Partners left disappointed after Hong Kong public hospitals bring back ban on delivery rooms to protect pregnant women amid Covid-19 surge. *South China Morning Post.* https://www.scmp.com/news/hong-kong/health-environment/article/3167720/partners-left-disappointed-after-hong-kong-public?module=inline&pgtype=article

Whitehead, K. (2020, February 25). Why Hong Kong panic buying happened: Herd mentality, the media, overreaction and distrust. *South China Morning Post.* https://www.scmp.com/lifestyle/health-wellness/article/3052101/why-hong-kong-panic-buying-happened-herd-mentality-media

Whitehead, K. (2022, March 1). How Covid-19 quarantine isolation in Hong Kong is hurting mental health amid reports of suicide attempts at Penny's Bay. *South China Morning Post.* https://www.scmp.com/lifestyle/health-wellness/article/3168650/how-covid-19-quarantine-isolation-hong-kong-hurting

Whitehead, K. (2023, February 9). Hong Kong's favourite Covid news tweeter Tripperhead wins official recognition and says the tweets will go on. *South China Morning Post.* https://www.scmp.com/lifestyle/health-wellness/article/3209477/hong-kongs-beloved-covid-news-tweeter-tripperhead-wins-official-recognition-and-says-tweets-will-go

Wong, M. (2021). The impacts of Covid-19 on foreign domestic workers in Hong Kong. *Asian Journal of Business Ethics, 10*(2), 357–370.

Wong, W. (2020, November 16). Anxiety, isolation among Hong Kong's elderly amid Covid-19 pandemic—and how you can help. *South China Morning Post.* https://www.scmp.com/news/hong-kong/society/article/3109932/anxiety-isolation-among-hong-kongs-elderly-amid-covid-19

Woodhouse, A. (2020, February 17). Hong Kong toilet roll heist underscores coronavirus panic-buying. *Financial Times.* https://www.ft.com/content/53e2de26-5146-11ea-90ad-25e377c0ee1f

World Health Organization. (2022a, March 2). *COVID-19 pandemic triggers 25% increase in prevalence of anxiety and depression worldwide* [Press release]. https://www.who.int/news/item/02-03-2022-covid-19-pandemic-triggers-25-increase-in-prevalence-of-anxiety-and-depression-worldwide

World Health Organization. (2022b, March 15). *Coronavirus disease (COVID-19): Pregnancy, childbirth and the postnatal period*. World Health Organization. https://www.who.int/news-room/questions-and-answers/item/coronavirus-disease-covid-19-pregnancy-and-childbirth

World Health Organization. (2002c, June 17). Mental health. https://www.who.int/news-room/fact-sheets/detail/mental-health-strengthening-our-response/

Xie, Y. J., Yuen, J. T. A. L., Lam, S., Zhang, D., Yan, L., & Bressington, D. (2021). Hong Kong nurses' stress level and post-traumatic stress disorder during the outbreak of COVID-19 and the associations with their daily lives. https://research.polyu.edu.hk/en/publications/hong-kong-nurses-stress-level-and-post-traumatic-stress-disorder-

Yau, C. (2022, March 29). Coronavirus: Show concern for family and friends, experts urge as Hong Kong suicide index hits 'crisis level' in Covid-19 fifth wave. *South China Morning Post*. https://www.scmp.com/news/hong-kong/article/3172319/coronavirus-show-concern-family-and-friends-experts-urge-hong-kong

Yeung, N., Huang, B., Lau, C. Y., & Lau, J. T. (2020). Feeling anxious amid the COVID-19 pandemic: Psychosocial correlates of anxiety symptoms among Filipina domestic helpers in Hong Kong. *International Journal of Environmental Research and Public Health*, *17*(21), 8102.

Yiu, W. (2023a, February 27). Tongue-tied from Covid pandemic: Masks, online lessons blamed for increase in Hong Kong children diagnosed with speech problems. *South China Morning Post*. https://www.scmp.com/news/hong-kong/education/article/3211609/tongue-tied-pandemic-masks-online-lessons-blamed-increase-hong-kong-children-diagnosed-speech

Yiu, W. (2023b, May 8). Number of Hong Kong students with mental health problems doubles in 4 years, with experts blaming 2019 social unrest and Covid. *South China Morning Post*. https://www.scmp.com/news/hong-kong/education/article/3219673/number-hong-kong-students-mental-health-problems-doubles-4-years-experts-blaming-2019-social-unrest

Yiu, W., & Zhao, Z. (2023, February 27). Covid's lost years: Hong Kong children bear the cost of missing school, as more are diagnosed with learning problems. *South China Morning Post*. https://www.scmp.com/news/hong-kong/education/article/3211593/covids-lost-years-hong-kong-children-bear-cost-missing-school-more-are-diagnosed-learning-problems

Zhao, Z. (2023, February 19). Rise in Hong Kong hiking mishaps and deaths as Covid-19 drove hordes outdoors, with many trekkers clueless, unprepared. *South China Morning Post*. https://www.scmp.com/news/hong-kong/health-environment/article/3210685/rise-hong-kong-hiking-mishaps-and-deaths-covid-19-drove-hordes-outdoors-many-trekkers-clueless

About the Author

Kate Whitehead is an award-winning journalist and author of two Hong Kong crime books, *After Suzie* and *Hong Kong Murders*. She is also a qualified psychotherapist with a special interest in the treatment of anxiety issues, stress, and trauma.

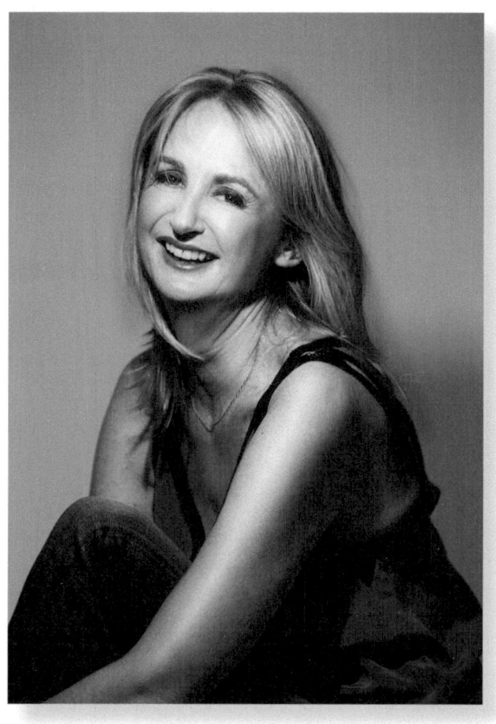